# Living with Multiple Sclerosis
## A Wellness Approach
### Second Edition

# Living with Multiple Sclerosis
## A Wellness Approach
### Second Edition

---

## George H. Kraft, M.D., MS
Director, Multiple Sclerosis Clinical Center
Director, Multiple Sclerosis Research and Training Center
University of Washington Medical Center
Professor, Rehabilitation Medicine
Adjunct Professor, Neurology
Seattle, Washington

## Marci Catanzaro, R.N., C.S.
Gerontological Nurse Practitioner
Primary Health Care Associates
Seattle, Washington

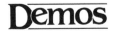

**Demos Medical Publishing, Inc., 386 Park Avenue South, New York, New York 10016**

*Library of Congress Cataloging-in-Publication Data*

Kraft, George H.
 Living with multiple sclerosis : a wellness approach/George H. Kraft, Marci
Catanzaro.–2nd ed.
  p. cm.
 Includes bibliographical references and index.
 ISBN 1-888799-26-9 (pbk.)
  1. Multiple sclerosis–Popular works. I. Catanzaro, Marci. II. Title.

RC377 .K73 2000
362.1'96834–dc21                                                    00-020502

Made in the United States of America

# Acknowledgments

Special credit and thanks to Pam Cavallo, Director of the Client & Community Services Department, for creating and nurturing the national teleconference program, and to Cindee McLaughlin, Senior Services Consultant, for her ongoing assistance with this project.

# Contents

# Foreword to the First Edition

How can someone who has a chronic disease like multiple sclerosis also be healthy? The answer is by choosing behaviors that promote health. The World Health Organization views health as the optimal level of function and well-being within the possible limitations imposed by a physical or mental impairment. As multiple sclerosis fluctuates or even progresses, the overall physical and emotional capacity can be nurtured, and improvement achieved within realistic goals. This broad and positive approach to health is also conceptualized as "wellness," with emphasis on those areas within our control, those opportunities to make thoughtful and informed choices to enhance our function, attitudes, and general sense of well-being. This approach not only has implications for the present, but can also impact long-term health. Cardiovascular fitness feels good today, but also reduces risk of heart attacks and stroke in later years. In order to choose wisely, it is necessary to be informed of the ramifications of various behaviors and activities. This book addresses the overall area of choices for wellness and related issues.

The first edition of this book was adapted from the question and answer portion of "Taking Control: Options to Maximize Your Health," a national teleconference produced by the National Multiple Sclerosis Society. This program won a silver national Health Information Award, and the Society is gratified that the response to the first edition of the book based on this program was so well received that it has now been updated and expanded in a new second edition.

A primary function of the Society is to provide information about multiple sclerosis (MS) to a variety of audiences, including people with MS, their families, health professionals, employers, and the general public. I am delighted that the valuable information provided by Drs. Kraft and Catanzaro to our teleconference participants is being shared with an even wider audience. It is critical for people with MS to maximize their health by reaching for even higher levels of physical and emotional wellness.

*Nancy J. Holland, Ed.D.*
*Vice President, Clinical Programs Department*
*National Multiple Sclerosis Society*

# Preface to the Second Edition

The first edition of this book was an outgrowth of questions raised during a national teleconference by people with multiple sclerosis (MS), their family members, and friends. Each day scientists learn more about the mechanisms that cause MS, ways of slowing the progression of the disease, and how to treat its symptoms. This second edition incorporates many of the recent developments in management of MS learned in the past few years, and new sections have been added. The value of a question and answer book, such as this one, is that the questions often remain the same. This book updates the answers. Questions have another purpose. They can serve as a study guide to learning more about MS. Ask these questions over and over as research produces greater insight and more complete answers. Ask questions of your health care provider, speakers at multiple sclerosis educational programs, the staff at the National Multiple Sclerosis Society, and anyone else whom you believe may have new answers to old questions. These questions may serve to stimulate your thinking and raise other questions about causes and treatment of MS and the management of symptoms.

No matter what new information is forthcoming about the causes and treatments of MS, successful living with this progressive neurologic disease depends on the person with disease. Taking control of your life in order to maximize your health is essential for each of us, whether or not we have MS. This book suggests some avenues for optimizing your health through exercise, nutrition, and emotional health. Use it as a jumping off point for putting together your own individualized program of wellness. Everyone needs a wellness program that addresses his or her individualized strengths and weaknesses. Consult your health care providers, nutritionist, therapist, and counselors. You are the most important person in maintaining your wellness.

We hope to bring a uniform perspective to this book. Initially, we worked together in the University of Washington Multiple Sclerosis Center when it was beginning. Presently, Dr. Kraft directs the Clinic, and Dr. Catanzaro sees community patients in private offices. We hope that this dual perspective will be useful to the patient with MS.

# CAUSE AND COURSE OF
# MULTIPLE SCLEROSIS

The cause of multiple sclerosis (MS) still eludes scientists, although more information is obtained every year. We do know many things about its etiology (cause) from epidemiologic and laboratory studies. For example, we know that MS is more common in the northern parts of the northern hemisphere and the southern parts of the southern hemisphere. It is much less common in tropical climates. We also know that people from certain genetic backgrounds have a much higher incidence of MS than others. For example, MS is far more common in people of northern European than African stock. Evidence points to the fact that it is where children grow up and spend the first half of the teen years—rather than where they live when the symptoms occur—that is associated with the likelihood of getting MS. Viral etiologies are suspected, but none has yet been proven. A popular line of thinking is that a frequent association with many childhood viruses—"increased viral load"— during the development of the immune system alters the immune system in genetically susceptible people, making it likely to go awry in adult years and attack the central nervous system (CNS) many years later.

Before the development of magnetic resonance imaging (MRI) and evoked potentials (EPs), such as visual, somatosensory, and brainstem evoked potentials, diagnosis was based on specific characteristics of the disease course. Abnormalities in several parts of the nervous system occurring over a period of time had to occur before the diagnosis could be made. Spinal fluid analysis often helped confirm the diagnosis. More recently, the MRI, EPs, and newer tests such as magnetic resonance spectroscopy (MRS) are enhancing the ability of clinicians to make the diagnosis early. In the past, it was not uncommon for a person to wait two or more years after the first symptoms appeared for a diagnosis to be made. With these new diagnostic tools, the diagnosis may now be made within days after the first onset of symptoms.

Although the course of MS is extremely variable, approximately 70 percent of people with the disease start with a relapsing and remitting course in which the remissions are complete and long in the early phases. At some point, exacerbations begin to occur more frequently and remissions are less complete. This course eventually tends to transform in most patients into what is known as a secondary progressive form, with a relatively steady worsening without the fluctuations seen earlier. Perhaps 5 percent to 10 percent of patients have a course that is progressive from onset (primary progressive MS). These patients tend to have a worse prognosis. They frequently are older men. Last, there is a mild form of the disease in which people may have a lifetime without significant problems, having just enough symptomatology and laboratory findings for the diagnosis to be made. It is unclear how many people have this form of MS; there actually may be more than medical practitioners suspect because symptomatology is minimal throughout the lives of most of these people.

# Pathology

*Q:* What exactly is multiple sclerosis?

*A:* Much has been learned about MS in the last few years. Until the present time, our understanding of the disease was based on pathologic studies and patterns of the disease course. Recent research using magnetic resonance spectroscopy (MRS) and more sophisticated microscopic studies, as well as immunology and frequent MRIs, have altered our understanding of MS. Although it is primarily a demyelinating disease—a disease in which the initial problem starts with the myelin coating of the nerve—we now know that the nerve fibers themselves may be pathologically altered, even when myelin is unaffected. Thus, the disease may be present in parts of the central nervous system other than just those showing demyelination.

*Q:* If I have an exacerbation, does that mean the disease is active?

*A:* This may be the most important area of new knowledge of MS. During the studies of Betaseron, and subsequently confirmed at the National Institutes of Health, an MRI was performed on some patients every several weeks. The results surprised the medical world. It appeared that exacerbations (new lesions developing) on MRI were seen far more frequently than clinical exacerbation occurred. Thus, for a person experiencing *clinical* exacerbations one or two times a year, detectable exacerbations were actually occurring as often as every one or two months. These exacerbations were occurring, however, in areas of more subtle clinical manifestation and were not noticed by the patient. Much of the brain is involved in memory, thought, emotion, and processing; exacerbations in these areas were not noticed as were exacerbations in pathology involving the eyes, arms and legs.

*Q:*   Why is this important to me?

*A:*   This is very important. These are the areas of the brain that represent "higher" functioning; these are the areas that make us human beings, not animals. They are vital areas to protect and explain the National MS Society's policy that once MS is diagnosed, it should be treated (see Appendix B).

# Disease Distribution

*Q:* Why is multiple sclerosis more prevalent in the North?

*A:* We know that in the northern hemisphere there is a higher prevalence of MS between 40° and 60° latitude. We also know that where people are born and reared, up to their mid-teen years, is more predictive of who gets MS than where they are living at the time symptoms appear. Although we do not know the reason for certain, many scientists suspect that it may relate to a higher incidence in colder climates of children playing together inside—and getting more viral infections, perhaps overloading or altering the immune system. There also is a genetic component: people of Northern European descent have a higher incidence of MS, and more of these people live in the North.

*Q:* Is multiple sclerosis more common in women?

*A:* Yes. In fact, MS is about twice as common in women as in men. We do not know why that is so, but we do know that other *autoimmune* diseases are also more common in women.

*Q:* What is an autoimmune disease?

*A:* An autoimmune disease is one in which the body's immune system attacks its own tissues. In MS the immune system attacks nerves in the central nervous system (brain and spinal cord). Other examples of autoimmune disease include rheumatoid arthritis and systemic lupus erythematosus.

*Q:* Do children get MS?

*A:* Yes, there are very rare but verified cases of MS in school-aged children. More typically, however, the disease has an onset between the ages of 15 and 50 years, with the average onset in the late twenties. Often people who are older when they are diagnosed with MS had their first symptoms many years before.

*Q:* Does MS affect one socioeconomic class more than another?

*A:* In the United States it appears that the disease is more common in higher socioeconomic groups. This may be related to the ethnicity of members of these groups. The most likely explanation is the known predisposition to MS because of genetic factors. Another part of the explanation may be that people in higher socioeconomic groups have better access to health care and are more likely to seek a diagnosis for neurologic symptoms. Without expensive testing, symptoms of MS may be attributed to other causes.

# Cause of Multiple Sclerosis

*Q:* Is MS caused by something in the environment?

*A:* The cause of MS is still not known. Various environmental factors, including specific viruses and toxins such as dental amalgam and organic solvents, have been suggested as possible causes, although there is absolutely no evidence that any of these agents cause the disease. Some studies have suggested that some combination of viral exposure in childhood may increase the likelihood of later developing MS. Many viruses have been studied, but none of them alone has been demonstrated to play a key role in the cause of the disease. No connection has been established between chemicals or toxins and the development of MS.

*Q:* Is MS a genetically inherited disease?

*A:* Some diseases, such as Duchenne's muscular dystrophy, are genetically inherited by the mendelian rules taught in high school biology. Multiple sclerosis is much more complex. The disease tends to occur more frequently in families than in the general population, but technically it is not considered a genetically inherited disease. People with certain genetic tissue markers are more likely to develop MS than people with other genetic markers. For example, because people of Scandinavian origin are much more likely to develop MS than people of African origin, there is probably a genetic *predisposition* to MS that is

7

related to how the body's immune system works. Genes alone do not determine who gets MS—some event must trigger the development of the disease, with the onset of the first symptoms occurring much later. We know from the study of identical twins, who have exactly the same genetic makeup, that it is possible for only one twin to develop MS, although the likelihood of a second twin developing the disease is greater than for siblings who are nonidentical.

*Q:* Is there a genetic test that is specific for multiple sclerosis?

*A:* No, there is no genetic test for MS. A variety of genetic *markers* have been associated with MS. However, not everyone with the disease has these markers, and not everyone who has these markers develops MS.

*Q:* How is the immune system related to MS?

*A:* The immune system is incredibly complex. Entire books have been written about it, and yet there is much to be learned. Very simply, T lymphocytes (a type of white blood cell) regulate the invasion of viruses and resist bacterial invasion and malignant cell changes. For reasons that we still do not understand, T lymphocytes play a key role in the destruction of myelin, behaving as if myelin were a foreign substance. Abnormal levels of *killer T cells* and *suppressor T cells* have been found in the blood and spinal fluid of people with MS, especially during an exacerbation. The immunology of MS is one of the most active areas of current research. Scientists may soon have answers to this important matter.

*Q:* Is there any relationship between AIDS and MS?

*A:* Both diseases involve the immune system. Beyond that there is no similarity. Basic research on how the immune system works and things that alter its function will contribute to our understanding of MS and other diseases that affect the immune system.

# Diagnosis

*Q:* What is required by most doctors to confirm a diagnosis of MS?

*A:* The diagnosis of MS continues to present challenges, although it is much easier than it was 10 to 15 years ago. The name *multiple sclerosis* indicates what is necessary to make a diagnosis—at least two (multiple) areas of myelin destruction of scarring (sclerosis) present in the central nervous system (brain and spinal cord) must be identified. In other words, *more than one area of the brain or spinal cord must be involved in the disease process*. Newer diagnostic techniques such as MRI scans and evoked potential studies can help identify areas of damaged myelin before they produce symptoms and can thus be helpful in identifying additional sites of pathology to confirm a diagnosis. In years past the diagnosis of definite MS took a longer time because these tests were not available to "look" into the central nervous system. As recently as 20 years ago, there was an average of approximately two years between the time a person consulted his or her physician with symptoms and when the diagnosis was made. That is why some people then were initially told they *possibly* or *probably* had MS. Even now, however, there are cases in which the diagnosis cannot be made with complete certainty. Because of the availability of effective immune-modulating drugs, diagnosis is even more important now than it was in the past.

*Q:* Are spinal fluid analysis and biopsy necessary to diagnosis MS?

*A:* Structural changes in the central nervous system can be seen on MRI scans, and physiologic changes in nerve conduction can be measured by visual, somatosensory, and brainstem auditory evoked potentials. Spinal fluid analysis can be useful to identify changes in protein content that are typically associated with MS. A biopsy would only be required if the lesions mimicked an abnormal growth that might be a tumor. Invasive tests, such as spinal tap and biopsy, have largely been replaced by MRI and evoked potential tests.

*Q:* How long does it take for MS to appear on an MRI?

*A:* Typically, by the time a person has the first symptoms of MS, an MRI will identify multiple lesions. However, in approximately five percent to seven percent of people with MS, the initial lesions are in the spinal cord—usually the cervical (neck) region—and not in the brain. Therefore, if a person with clinically suspected MS has a normal brain MRI, an MRI of the spinal cord should be done; the MRI must be taken of the most likely affected portion of the central nervous system.

*Q:* What disorders mimic MS?

*A:* Many abnormalities of the brain or spinal cord can cause symptoms similar to those of MS. Vascular problems such as mild strokes can mimic MS. Metabolic disorders such as vitamin B deficiencies or diabetes mellitus can affect the central nervous system. Nerves can be trapped between muscles or bones, producing symptoms of numbness, tingling, and weakness. Infections, tumors, and collagen diseases such as lupus erythematosus can produce a clinical picture similar to that of MS. Emotional problems may also produce symptoms that can be confused with MS.

*Q:* Should people who were diagnosed with MS before magnetic resonance imaging (MRI) and evoked potentials were available have these tests now?

*A:* The advent of new technology has made the diagnosis of MS easier, faster, and more accurate. There probably is no need to apply this new technology to confirm the diagnosis if you have already been diagnosed with definite MS based on strict clinical criteria and the disease has taken the classic disease course (exacerbation followed by remission). There may, however, be reason to do such testing if it is desired to assess the amount of disease present or to use such information in the plan to implement disease-modifying therapies such as Avonex, Betaseron, or Copaxone. Also, if your diagnosis is "probable" or "possible" MS, you will want to have these newer tests performed in order to establish a firm diagnosis. You also may want these tests if there is reason to suspect that you have developed another disorder of the nervous system. For example, people with MS can also get a herniated disc or have a stroke, and the tests can be useful in determining the cause of the new symptoms.

*Q:* Why are more cases of MS being diagnosed now?

*A:* Several factors contribute to the apparently increased incidence of MS. First, we now have much more sophisticated diagnostic capabilities. The MRI scan and electrophysiologic tests help to identify demyelinated areas in the brain and spinal cord so that physicians can be more certain of the diagnosis earlier in the course of the disease. Second, there was a long period in the history of medicine during which nothing could be done to alter the course of MS, so many people were not told their diagnosis. Physicians are much more likely to tell people that they have MS now because we have immune-modifying drugs that reduce the frequency and severity of exacerbations and other medications to treat its symptoms.

# Disease Course

*Q:* How do you know whether you have the *relapsing-remitting* or *progressive type* of MS?

*A:* In general, an exacerbating and remitting course of MS is just that—symptoms flare up or worsen or new symptoms appear and then get at least somewhat better. This is the most common type of MS. In primary progressive MS, the disease simply moves steadily ahead from the onset and the person's condition continues to worsen. Approximately 70 percent of people with MS start out having exacerbating and remitting disease. Later in the course of the disease, remissions may become less complete, and there is more and more residual disability. After many years, many people no longer have exacerbations and remissions, and the disease then follows a secondary progressive course.

*Q:* Why do remissions occur?

*A:* The earliest stage of an attack is thought to be swelling (edema). A local reaction takes place, much like what you see when you injure your skin. The surrounding area becomes inflamed and swollen, and nerve conduction may be blocked. If this persists or becomes more severe, myelin (the coating or "insulation" of a nerve) may be destroyed. However, it may not progress to this stage, and the inflammation may gradually disappear. As the inflammatory response around an affected area diminishes, symptoms become less severe. A great deal of myelin needs to be damaged and replaced by scar tissue before symptoms become permanent.

*Q:* What can trigger an exacerbation?
*A:* The unpredictable nature of MS causes us to search for something that causes a worsening of symptoms. Emotional stress, immunizations, infections and other illnesses, changes in the weather, and trauma have all been held responsible for causing exacerbations. However, the scientific evidence does not support any theories that these factors consistently cause problems for people with MS. People with MS do, however, become worse with fever brought on by infection—often a urinary tract infection. Symptoms improve with successful treatment of the infection. Many call this a "pseudoexacerbation."

*Q:* Can poor nutrition trigger an episode?
*A:* Poor nutrition has many long-term effects. However, there is no evidence that it is directly associated with an exacerbation of MS.

*Q:* Does natural adrenaline associated with stress prevent exacerbations?
*A:* That is a very good question. There is a classic observation that during the Gulf War in 1991, when the Israelis were under attack by Iraqi missiles, the incidence of MS exacerbations declined, suggesting that stress offered a protection from exacerbations. When we are under a lot of stress, our bodies normally produce high levels of adrenal corticoids, which are natural substances similar to the drugs used to treat exacerbations of MS. People with MS often have no problems during brief high-stress periods; however, some patients consistently become worse when they are under stress. When the stressful period is over, a rapid decrease in cortisol levels occurs, and some people have an exacerbation. Thus, although evidence of the effect of acute stress in producing exacerbations is mixed, there is general agreement that long-standing chronic stress is detrimental to people with MS.

*Q:* What wellness therapies are most likely to bring about a remission?
*A:* Unfortunately, we do not understand enough about the basic pathophysiology of exacerbations and remissions to answer that

question. Certainly such things as keeping yourself in optimal health are a critical part of dealing with MS. Following a well-balanced diet, getting an adequate amount of sleep, and avoiding infectious diseases are all important. Bladder or lung infections can raise body temperature and make symptoms temporarily worse, but there is no evidence that they affect the long-term course of MS.

*Q:* Can exercise change the course of MS?

*A:* No. Exercise in and of itself does not alter the course of MS. Studies have, however, shown that both resistive exercise (lifting weights) and aerobic exercise (e.g., using an exercise bicycle) can produce some degree of positive benefit in people with MS. Because a person with MS may be weaker to start with, the improvement in strength that results from exercise may actually improve function considerably. Because most people with MS are sensitive to heat, it is important to try to keep body temperature from rising too much during exercise.

*Q:* Are there specific factors that determine how fast MS will progress?

*A:* The best estimates we have are really "guesstimates" as to the future. Certain onset patterns can help to predict where MS will be 5, 10, or 15 years later. In general, those who have little disability 5 years after onset have a better long-term *prognosis* (future predictions) than those who are fairly disabled at that time. People whose MS started with ataxia (movement problems or tremor) or weakness tend to have a poorer prognosis than do those whose MS started with sensory symptoms. An absence of initial remission is also a poor prognostic sign.

*Q:* If I am doing okay, do I need treatment?

*A:* Recent research has markedly altered our understanding of MS. We now know that for every clinical (noticeable) exacerbation, there will probably have been a number of silent or unnoticed exacerbations. Thus, the disease is probably active, even though it may not seem so. For this reason, the National Multiple Sclerosis Society has recommended treatment with an immune-modulating medication once the diagnosis has been established. (For more on this, see Section I on pathology and Appendix B).

# SYMPTOM MANAGEMENT

It is said that we are known by the company we keep. Similarly, multiple sclerosis is a disease known by its symptoms.

A person with MS does not typically think of the nerve damage and demyelination in central nervous tissue that occurs, but rather thinks of the symptoms that these "short circuits" produce. A person with MS will more likely think about weakness, fatigue, tingling, or spasticity. Because MS occurs at various sites in the brain and spinal cord, the longer the pathway that the nerve impulse must take, the more likely it is that nerve function will be interrupted and symptoms will occur. For example, the nerves to the bladder come from the spinal cord just below the nerves to the lower legs. Because of their distance from the brain, and the probability that nerve impulses from the brain—having to traverse so long a path—will likely encounter an area of disease, these two areas have the highest probability of being clinically affected. People with MS know the frequency of symptoms in these areas.

Although the "bad news" is that the bladder and lower legs are frequently affected in people with MS, the "good news" is that there are many things that can be done about these symptoms. Various types of medications and treatments are useful for people with bladder dysfunction, and exercise and bracing can help people with ankle and foot weakness.

Because of the interruption in the central nervous system, other symptoms such as fatigue, balance problems, temperature sensitivity, and muscle spasms may also occur. Even though the damaged nerves causing these problems cannot be repaired, there are steps that can be taken—both medical and nonmedical—to alleviate many of the symptoms produced by interruption of these nerve pathways. Similar types of nerve dysfunction can also affect the sensory pathways and produce various types of pain.

Many therapies can help people who have problems caused by these interrupted nerve pathways; these therapies are discussed in this section and the following three sections (Wellness Management, Emotional Health, and Disease Treatments). It should also be remembered that MS does not necessarily occur in isolation. People with MS can develop other problems, such as arthritis in the joints or disc problems in the back, which may interact with the symptoms of MS to make diagnosis and management very difficult. In this section we also answer some questions on this matter.

# Balance

---

*Q:* What can be done to improve balance and coordination?

*A:* A physical therapist can work with someone who is experiencing problems with balance. Some exercises, such as Frenkel's repetitive placement exercises, will improve balance and coordination to some degree. However, the most practical and effective treatment in most cases is to use a walker. If a person is strong but has poor balance, a walker can provide the extra amount of stability needed to allow safe walking. If balance is only mildly impaired, using a cane may be sufficient to allow safe walking. If weakness is present in addition to balance problems, or if the balance problem is severe, a scooter or wheelchair may be required.

*Q:* What treatments or strategies can be used to treat dizziness or vertigo?

*A:* Dizziness or vertigo may be caused by demyelination of parts of the brain that are responsible for balance and coordination. Sometimes a plaque on the floor of the fluid-filled spaces in the brain (ventricles) can cause dizziness. These symptoms are very difficult to treat. Sometimes dizziness and vertigo are related to position, and the person can learn to get up slowly and avoid rapid movement of the head. Medications to treat vertigo are sometimes helpful. Special attention must be paid to drugs used to treat other symptoms of MS, some of which have effects on the brain that may contribute to feelings of light-headedness and dizziness. One must be sure that the symptoms are not side effects of some other medication.

# Bladder and Bowel

*Q:* What causes bladder control problems in some people with MS?

*A:* Bladder problems are very common and are caused by damage in parts of the brain or spinal cord. Different types of bladder problems can occur in MS. One type occurs when the bladder does not empty completely, because the simultaneous bladder contraction and sphincter (exit valve) relaxation that allows urine to be expelled does not function as it should. This is known as bladder "dyssynergia" and can result in leakage of urine and a tendency to urinary tract infections. A second type of problem occurs when the bladder is hyperactive and contracts in response to a small amount of urine. This is associated with incontinence. Rarely is the problem due only to a lack of strength of bladder contraction, which results in some urine remaining in the bladder.

*Q:* How do you know what kind of bladder problem MS is causing?

*A:* It is not always possible to tell the kind of bladder dysfunction by signs and symptoms alone. The end result of a bladder that does not empty completely, or one that empties too often, is urinary frequency and incontinence. It is important to have the problem assessed by a practitioner who understands the neurologic causes of bladder dysfunction. Sometimes people with MS have a combination of problems with the urinary sphincter and bladder contraction.

*Q:*  What diagnostic tests need to be done to assess bladder problems?

*A:*  Measuring the amount of urine left in the bladder after a person empties his or her bladder (postvoid residual, or PVR) will show if the bladder is emptying completely. A bladder filling test (cystometrogram) can show how sensitive the bladder is to stretching as it fills and the person's ability to suppress the urge to void. Sometimes it is also necessary to study the sphincter muscles with electromyography. A cystoscopy is necessary when bladder stones or pathology of the bladder lining is suspected.

*Q:*  How can bladder problems be managed?

*A:*  The key to managing bladder problems is understanding the neurologic status of the bladder and the relationship between fluid intake and a full bladder. A three-day diary of fluid intake, the time and quantity of urine voided, and episodes of leaking urine is important in establishing a treatment program for bladder problems. Intervention strategies may include timing fluid intake and voiding by the clock rather than waiting for urgency to occur. Protective undergarments can be used if incontinence continues to be a problem. Medications can be used to decrease the hypersensitivity of the bladder to filling or to relax a spastic sphincter. A new medicine—DDAVP—can be used to slow the kidney's production of urine for a period of several hours, thus allowing a person with a tendency to incontinence to be continent for many hours and to comfortably engage in protracted social activities or to sleep through the night. Intermittent self-catheterization is a strategy that works for many people, both in relieving symptoms and in preventing potentially serious complications. The benefit of an indwelling catheter sometimes outweighs the increased risk of infections and stone formation. Surgical interventions are a last resort and are rarely indicated.

*Q:*  Are there specific exercises to help manage bladder problems?

*A:*  Muscles in the floor of the pelvis contribute to the ability to store urine in the bladder until it is appropriate to urinate. It is not uncommon for women to have weak muscles in the floor of the pelvis. Kegel exercises, in which these muscles are consciously contracted about 200 times a day, can strengthen them and decrease the type of incontinence that occurs when bladder pressure exceeds sphincter contraction, such as during coughing or sneezing. Biofeedback is also helpful in learning how to exercise the pelvic floor muscles. Abdominal muscles help empty the bladder, and they can also be strengthened through exercise.

*Q:*   Is autonomic dysreflexia a real threat to people with MS?

*A:*   Autonomic dysreflexia occurs when there is a complete transection of the spinal cord above the midthoracic level. When this occurs, the stretched bladder or rectum stimulates the autonomic nervous system and messages from the brain to suppress dangerously elevated blood pressure and other physiologic responses cannot get past the spinal cord injury. It is very rare for someone with MS to have plaques that result in complete functional interruption of the spinal cord at this level.

*Q:*   Is acupuncture helpful for MS-related bladder problems?

*A:*   There is much about acupuncture that we do not clearly understand. It seems to be beneficial for some symptoms of MS, particularly pain-related symptoms. There is no evidence that acupuncture alters bladder function in MS in the long term.

*Q:*   What can be done about bowel problems in MS?

*A:*   Normal bowel movements require adequate fluid and fiber in the diet to maintain a soft consistency of stool. The ability to contract and relax the anal sphincter at will is also necessary. A high-fiber diet, at least 48 ounces of fluid a day, and a regular time for having a bowel movement are essential components of a bowel management program. Eating a breakfast that includes a warm liquid capitalizes on the natural gastrocolic reflex and encourages bowel emptying at a predictable time. Occasionally it is necessary to add a suppository to a bowel program. The regular use of laxatives is rarely indicated.

# Fatigue

*Q:* Does everyone who has MS experience fatigue?

*A:* Fatigue is the most common symptom in MS, although rarely is it the most severe. The exact cause of MS fatigue is not known, but it is thought to be related to myelin damage as well as to secondary weakness of muscles. It may also be caused by disease activity. Muscle weakness may result in increased energy requirements to carry out the common activities of daily living. Depression may also result in fatigue. Pain or stress can alter sleep patterns, thus producing another type of fatigue from inadequate sleep. The type of fatigue experienced by persons with MS appears to be unique to the disorder and is not just an extreme form of the "tiredness" we all feel from time to time.

*Q:* When symptoms increase in intensity during the day, is it better to continue at the current pace or slack off?

*A:* A person with MS who has fatigue in the afternoon or after sustained activity should definitely take a period of rest. Rest can improve the ability to function during the remainder of the day.

*Q:* How can a physiatrist help with fatigue?

*A:* A physiatrist is a physician who has specialized in rehabilitation. Much of what is involved in the management of MS is rehabilitation. For example, the physiatrist can help prevent contractures and complications, which would result in the need for more energy for the person to carry out activities of daily living. The physiatrist can also prescribe equipment that conserves energy and lessens fatigue.

*Q:* How can one distinguish between fatigue that is necessary to build stamina and fatigue that could cause an exacerbation of MS?

*A:* Evidence from recent research studies indicates that fatigue that results from exercise will not produce an exacerbation. The negative aspect of fatigue in the person with MS is that in some people—but probably very few—the feeling of tiredness may be prolonged to the point that it makes the benefits of exercise not worth the trade-off. However, muscle fatigue is an essential part of obtaining maximal benefit from exercise. The ideal is to get enough exercise of muscles without excessive tiredness or central fatigue. An individual's prescription for exercise can balance these elements. Recent research studies show that both aerobic (endurance) and resistive (weight lifting) exercise can safely help most people with MS to perform and feel better.

*Q:* Why do symptoms of MS get worse with exercise?

*A:* They usually don't. However, there is a temperature at which nerve conduction takes place most efficiently. When there is demyelination of nerve fibers in the spinal cord or brain, the sensitivity to elevation in temperature is greater than in unaffected, normally myelinated nerve fibers. Excessive exercise can increase core body temperature, which may result in impaired nerve conduction and increase fatigue or temporarily worsen other symptoms.

*Q:* What strategies can be used to reduce overheating during exercise?

*A:* Pay attention to your environment. Exercise in a cool room with low humidity or in the shade. Low humidity increases evaporation of perspiration. Eat ice chips while exercising. A commercially available cooling vest can also keep core body temperature from increasing during exercise.

*Q:* Are there any medications that reduce fatigue?

*A:* Amantadine (Symmetrel®) is the drug of choice in treating the fatigue associated with MS. It is a safe medication that is helpful in approximately one third of people with MS. Pemoline (Cylert®), a type of stimulant, may be helpful for people who do not respond to amantadine. 4-aminopyridine (4-AP) can reduce symptoms of MS in general, including fatigue. This drug, however, appears to be most effective in people whose symptoms are exacerbated when they become hot, and it is not yet available in the United States because of problems with safety. Studies are exploring ways to modify the peripheral and central effects of fatigue.

*Q:*   What is the relationship between fatigue and depression in MS?

*A:*   Depression in MS may be "organic," resulting from demyelination in the brain. It also may be "reactive," a consequence of the personal loss brought about by MS. Depression interferes with normal eating and sleeping patterns and generally makes people tired. Antidepressant medications and psychological counseling are helpful ways to manage the fatigue that results from depression.

# Tremor and Spasms

*Q:* Is there any treatment for tremor?

*A:* Severe tremor is probably the most difficult MS-related problem to treat. Currently there is no effective nonsurgical treatment for severe tremor. For mild tremors, one treatment that has essentially no side effects is the use of a weight on an extremity to increase its mass, and thus reduce the extent of the tremor. For example, a 3–5 pound weight can be strapped to the wrist to assist in eating or self-care. Several medications, such as propranolol or isoniazid, have also been reported to help and can be tried, although our experience with these drugs has generally been disappointing. Surgical treatments are sometimes used for severe tremor. A technique called surgical thalamotomy has been used to give some relief of severe tremor, although it may have limits in the duration of effectiveness and cannot be used for tremor of the head or body. A new surgical technique called *deep brain stimulation* is being studied and may offer some help to MS patients with severe tremor.

*Q:* What exercises can be done to decrease leg tremor when standing?

*A:* Shaking of the legs may be due to spasticity, ataxia, or muscle weakness. Management depends on which of these problems is causing the symptom. Stretching a tight muscle can help reduce the stretch reflex in a spastic muscle and allow better joint position. Consequently, less muscle energy is required to stand, and leg shaking may be reduced.

Pharmacologic treatment is almost always also indicated, with baclofen (Lioresal®) and tizanidine (Zanaflex®) generally the most effective medications. Too much baclofen should be avoided because it may produce additional weakness (small amounts of spasticity can actually enhance standing in weak muscles). Too much tizanidine and baclofen may cause sleepiness. If the problem is ataxia, ankle weights may also reduce shaking, much in the same way that wrist weights can reduce upper limb ataxia. Severe leg tremor will require the use of a walker or wheelchair.

*Q:* What can be done about the lumps or bumps in muscle fibers associated with muscle spasms?

*A:* Multiple sclerosis can produce spasms in muscles, but in general the whole muscle becomes tight and reflexes become exaggerated. There is a condition known as myofascial pain, or fibrosis, which causes muscle pain. This can cause "lumps" in muscles so that they feel like ropes when rubbed or palpated. There is no laboratory test to diagnose fibrositis. Lumps and bumps in muscles are more likely to be related to fibrositic problems than to MS.

*Q:* What are the current recommendations for managing nighttime muscle spasms?

*A:* Spasms can be related to MS or may be simple muscle cramps identical to those that occur in people without MS. Multiple sclerosis can increase spasticity in muscles, and certain positions in bed can trigger this spasticity. There are two approaches to management. One is to stretch the affected muscle before bedtime so that the stretch reflex of that muscle will not be set off by a small amount of movement. The second is to use a pharmacologic agent such as baclofen (Lioresal®) or tizanidine (Zanaflex®) to treat spasticity. Many physicians believe that tizanidine is the better medication because it seems to have more effect on nocturnal spasms and also produces somnolence. A combination of stretching exercises, physical therapy, and pharmacologic intervention may be necessary to control nighttime muscle spasms.

*Q:* What nonpharmacologic strategies can be used to deal with painful spasms?

*A:* Physical medicine interventions are the best strategies for alleviating painful muscle spasms. Stretching and other exercises can help ameliorate these symptoms. Physicians who specialize in physical medicine and rehabilitation (physiatrists) and physical therapists can assess the problem and prescribe strategies specific to each individual.

*Q:*  What can you tell us about myoclonic jerks?

*A:*  Myoclonic jerks and twitches commonly occur as an individual falls asleep; they do not require intervention. If the jerks become a serious problem, it may be necessary to rule out seizures. Drugs that are used to treat myoclonic epilepsy can be tried. A neurologist or physiatrist can accurately diagnose the problem and prescribe the correct pharmacologic intervention.

*Q:*  What medications are used to treat spasms in MS?

*A:*  Oral baclofen is the initial drug of choice for the pharmacologic treatment of spasticity in MS. Possible side effects of this medication include additional muscle weakness, drowsiness, and fatigue. Nausea is a potential side effect that can be avoided by taking the medication with food. Some patients benefit from high doses of baclofen but experience too many side effects. If spasticity is primarily limited to the lower limbs, a small catheter can be placed in the spinal canal and connected to a small implanted pump that administers baclofen directly to the spinal cord. This form of administration—called a baclofen pump—is very effective for patients who have spasticity in the lower limbs and cannot tolerate high doses of oral baclofen. A new drug that does not have the muscle weakening side effect of baclofen is tizanidine. This medication needs to be increased in the system gradually and very slowly because it may produce sleepiness. Other drugs that may be used for spasticity include dantrolene sodium (Dantrium®) and diazepam (Valium®). Some patients benefit from a regimen of combination therapy.

*Q:*  Are new antiinflammatory drugs helpful for muscle spasms?

*A:*  No. Antiinflammatory drugs are not effective for muscle spasms. These drugs, which include aspirin, corticosteroids, and nonsteroidal antiinflammatories (NSAIDs), are used to treat inflammation of tissue, such as that which occurs in arthritis; intravenous corticosteroids are indicated to treat MS exacerbations.

# Pain

---

*Q:* How prevalent is pain with MS?

*A:* Pain is not an uncommon problem in people with MS, and when it is severe, it can be among the most difficult symptoms to treat. Pain may result from a variety of problems. It often results because muscles become fatigued and stretched when they are used to compensate for muscles that have been weakened by MS. Muscle spasms can also cause pain. People with MS may also experience a kind of pain—called neuropathic or central pain—that results from faulty nerve signals produced by initiation of nerves by MS lesions in the spinal cord or brain. This typically is an intermittent, very sharp "stabbing" pain. The damaged area of the spinal cord or brain irritates nerve and incorrectly interprets pain signals as coming from another part of the body. Sometimes normal touching of skin is interpreted as pain because of the mixed-up messages occurring in the central nervous system. People with MS can develop other painful health conditions as well. Never assume that new pain is "just my MS"—have it evaluated by your health care provider.

*Q:* What causes musculoskeletal pain?

*A:* A person with MS is just as vulnerable as anyone else to having pain from muscles, tendons, joints, and bones. This types of pain can be differentiated from neuropathic pain because it is more steady and achy. A person with MS may actually have a greater tendency for these types of pain because they may not have normal joint range and muscle strength.

*Q:* Why is back pain so common in MS?

*A:* Back pain is a major health care problem in this country. It is the single most common cause of missed work for people who do not have MS. Because weakened muscles in the back and abdomen are often a factor in back pain, the best treatment for most cases of acute or chronic back pain is exercise. Unfortunately, people with MS do not always have the ability to generate sufficient intramuscular tension necessary to produce muscular hypertrophy, or the endurance to do sufficient aerobic exercise. Building up the muscles in the back and abdomen to stabilize the back may not be possible. Wearing a corset during periods of acute back strain can be an effective way to compensate for weakened muscles.

*Q:* Can specific exercises help to control pain?

*A:* Pain that results from muscle imbalance can effectively be treated by exercise in some people with MS. Each person will require careful evaluation by a knowledgeable health care provider, such as a physiatrist or a physical therapist, to determine what muscles are weak and which are compensating. An individualized exercise program can be prescribed based on that information. Exercise should also help to decrease spasticity and soreness of those muscles.

*Q:* What drugs can be used to relieve excruciating pain?

*A:* The most disturbing pain in MS is that from damage to nerves in the central nervous system resulting from MS lesions. It cannot be alleviated by the usual pain-relieving drugs (e.g., aspirin or narcotics) because those medications do not address the central issue of what is causing the pain. Some of the drugs used to treat seizures, such as carbamazepine (Tegretol®), gabapentin (Neurontin®), phenytoin (Dilantin®), or divalproex sodium (Depakote®) are often effective in treating this central pain, as is a common antidepressant, amitriptyline (Elavil®)

*Q:* How can chronic pain be managed without drugs?

*A:* Relaxation techniques such as progressive relaxation, meditation, and deep breathing can contribute to the management of chronic pain. Biofeedback can also be used to learn ways to relax muscle groups that are causing pain. Many people have found that massage and chiropractic treatments are helpful in relieving muscle pains. Application of a warm moist cloth to an area that feels as if it is burning may stop the burning sensation for several hours. The application of ice to painful muscles for brief periods of time decreases pain. The transcutaneous electrical nerve stimulator (TENS) may also relieve pain. Hydrotherapy is also useful in relieving some kinds of pain in MS. Some patients obtain relief from acupuncture.

*Q:*  If a warm cloth helps relieve tingling, would a heating pad work?

*A:*  Something about moist heat for 10 to 15 minutes really does help. However, the danger of using a heating pad is that if it is used for too long, there is a much greater danger of burning skin that already has some changes in sensation and may not perceive that the heating pad is becoming too hot. In addition, many MS patients are very sensitive to heat. The use of a heating pad is not advised.

*Q:*  Can anything be done to minimize skin sensitivity?

*A:*  Skin sensitivity in MS usually results from some damage to the sensory pathways, which makes them overrespond to normal stimuli. Often sensitivity is more pronounced with light touch. Wearing clothing that is very loose is more comfortable than garments that fit snugly. If the problem is disabling, certain drugs used to treat seizures may decrease the sensitivity.

*Q:*  What information is available for people with MS who suffer from headaches.

*A:*  A person with MS can develop every other type of medical problem experienced by anyone else. Someone with headaches should consult a health care practitioner to determine whether the headaches are related to something other than MS (e.g., headaches caused by degenerative changes in the cervical spine or migraine headaches). Headaches are not related to MS and can be effectively treated.

# Weakness

*Q:* Can exercises strengthen muscles in MS?

*A:* Yes, Resistive, strength-building exercises can often increase strength just enough to improve functions. For a more detailed answer, see pages 46–47 on Exercise.

*Q:* What is the status of the use of electronic devices to stimulate the limbs?

*A:* A person with MS has the type of weakness that benefits from electrical stimulation of muscle (actually, it is not the "muscle" that is stimulated, but the tips of the nerves as they enter the muscle; for convenience, we refer to it as "muscle stimulation"). Consequently, those characteristics may make electrical stimulation techniques more widely used in the future. MS lesions are in the central nervous system—the brain and spinal cord. The peripheral nerves, which go from the spinal cord to the muscles in the limbs, are unaffected by MS. Muscles may be weak because the electrical signals cannot get through the central nervous system. Techniques that give messages directly to the peripheral nervous system have the potential for a very good treatment outcome. In some cases electrical stimulation is superior to bracing for weak muscles that cause foot drop.

*Q:* Can electrical stimulation strengthen muscles?

*A:* There is some evidence that electrical stimulation combined with voluntary exercise will produce more impressive hypertrophy (bulking up) of muscles in MS than either technique alone. The upper motor neurons of the brain and spinal cord are impaired in MS and electrical stimulation can, in a sense, substitute for a person's own activation of the brain to provide stimulation for peripheral nerves.

# Memory Difficulties
## and Other Cognitive Problems

*Q:* How many people with MS have memory loss?

*A:* No one knows exactly how many people actually have MS, let alone how many of those people have which symptoms. We at the University of Washington in Seattle and others are currently researching the matter. Memory problems are certainly a major concern for many people with MS. Studies have estimated that as few as 10 percent or as many as 90 percent of people with MS have some degree of memory impairment, usually in what is referred to as "short-term" memory. The majority of people with cognitive dysfunction continue to function without significant difficulty.

*Q:* What kind of memory is affected by MS?

*A:* There are two aspects to memory. One is the ability to remember things immediately—the type of memory necessary to acquire new information. The second component of memory is the ability to retrieve stored information. It has been assumed that people with MS have difficulty retrieving information, but newer information suggests that they may also have problems acquiring information. The parts of memory that are affected by the disease are being studied, but it will be a few years before good data are available.

*Q:* What causes memory loss in someone with MS?

*A:* Most commonly, memory problems are a result of actual structural damage from demyelination and axon loss within the brain. It should be remembered that recent research has shown that for every clinical or physical exacerbation, there may be as many as six or more episodes of disease flareup in the brain. Magnetic resonance imaging of brains taken every few weeks demonstrate much more disease activity than we had suspected on physical examination. The areas of brain affected probably are involved with memory, emotion, and other nonphysical aspects of life, so it should not be surprising that memory problems are common. However, there may be some other cause of memory problems as well. Memory impairment may be related to the side effects of drugs or the effects of stress. Sometimes MS is used as an excuse for being unable to remember things that someone without the disease cannot remember either! Short-term memory impairment is often a result of not paying attention to the content in the first place. (Teenagers and spouses often experience this type of memory impairment!)

*Q:* Is there an exercise or a special diet or vitamin that improves memory?

*A:* Although fish has been claimed to be "brain food," there is no universally accepted evidence that fish or any other food or dietary supplement improves memory. Ginkgo biloba and some prescription medicines have been touted as helpful by some clinicians. Ginkgo biloba interacts with many prescription drugs, so it is a good idea to check with your pharmacist before adding it to other herbs and prescription drugs. However, there are strategies to help improve memory, such as using associations to learn new material. Speech therapists are experts in helping MS patients learn compensating techniques. Libraries and bookstores have many self-help guides to improving memory.

*Q:* Do plasma infusions help memory loss and poor concentration?

*A:* Plasma infusions, or plasmapheresis, do not improve memory loss or poor concentration that is caused by destruction of myelin in the central nervous system, although this treatment is being researched for controlling progression of the disease itself. However, memory problems also may be caused by the side effects of medications used to treat spasticity, pain, or other symptoms in MS. Therefore, a person with poor memory who is taking medications should make sure that the problem is not a side effect of the drugs.

*Q:* Are there cognitive skills in addition to memory that may be impaired with MS?

*A:* Cognitive skills include attention, learning, memory, language, and thought. Demyelination and axon damage of areas of the brain that control these functions can cause problems in any of these areas. Much of the brain is devoted to the "higher functions," and it is to be expected that cognitive impairment may be a problem for some people with MS. That being said, it is not wise to attribute problems with remembering, planning, thinking ahead, or judgment to demyelination without investigation. These problems often result from the side effects of drugs, stress, or even other diseases, including vascular disease, diabetes, lung or heart disease, or nutritional deficiencies. Neuropsychological testing is one means to help analyze the difficulty.

# Communication Disorders:
# Hearing, Speech, and Vision

*Q:*  Is hearing loss normal with MS?

*A:*  No. However, multiple sclerosis can cause inflammation, blocks of nerve conduction, and demyelination in many parts of the central nervous system (CNS), including the brainstem, the area in which the acoustic nerve arises. When this occurs, the resultant ringing in the ears and loss of hearing can be difficult to treat. Intravenous (IV) corticosteroids such as methylprednisolone may help during an acute exacerbation, but they will not help a chronic problem.

*Q:*  Can speech therapy help someone whose speech is affected by MS?

*A:*  The most common cause of speech problems in MS is due to an impairment in the muscles that are needed for speaking. Speech may become slurred and difficult to understand. Speech therapists use a variety of techniques that may improve communication, although the problem cannot be cured. Another problem arises when chest muscles are weak and the person's voice is soft because he cannot get enough air behind it. Personal amplifier systems are inexpensive and work well to overcome this problem.

*Q:*  What vision problems can affect people with MS?

*A:*  Multiple sclerosis may affect the optic nerve (actually an extension of the brain) to the eye, which results in some impairment in vision; this is called optic neuritis. People often describe this as having "blind spots" or "like looking through a lace curtain." Currently, the most effective treatment for damage to the optic nerve is intravenous corticosteroids used for an acute exacerbation. Fortunately, visual problems of this type are usually self-limited and may improve in time. Some people experience double vision because of eye muscle weakness. Unfortunately, double vision in MS is usually dynamic—it changes too rapidly for a prism in eyeglasses to be effective. Wearing a patch over one eye stops double vision. It is important to switch the patch from one eye to the other on a regular basis or the patched eye will develop reduced vision.

*Q:* What communication aids are available when a person is unable to speak and has limited use of her hands and head.

*A:* The technology in nonvocal communication is constantly improving. There are a variety of communicators that actually speak or display a printed message based on the individual's ability to spell out words or to recognize words on a board. Those communication systems can interface with very simple on-off switches. Consultation with a speech pathologist and a bioengineer can often solve communication problems.

*Q:* Do insurance companies pay for communicators?

*A:* Insurance companies often do not cover communication devices. There is incredible pressure from society to reduce the amount of money spent on health care. People with diseases such as MS want sophisticated medical care, but society seems unwilling to pay for it. Technology is advancing, but it is very expensive. Managed care is having an adverse effect on the provision of sophisticated technology to help people with disabilities. It is important to contact policymakers in the House of Representatives and the Senate, on both the national and the state levels, as well as policymakers in insurance companies, to remind them not to neglect the needs of disabled people in the health care system.

# The Effect of Temperature on Symptoms

*Q:* Can heat make MS worse?

*A:* Heat probably does not make MS worse in the long term. However, when the core body temperature is raised, fatigue and other symptoms become more apparent in most, but not all, people with MS. This is a short-term effect, and symptoms abate when temperature returns to normal. A rise in core body temperature impairs nerve conduction in demyelinated nerves. The combined effect of damaged myelin and heat contributes to the worsening of symptoms. It is important for people who are sensitive to heat to stay in a cool environment with low humidity.

*Q:* How can core body temperature be kept down?

*A:* Stay in a cool environment with low humidity. However, in many climates that is easier said than done. A cool environment can be achieved through air conditioning. If your home is not air conditioned, you can legitimately deduct it from income tax as a medical expense. Spend time in shopping malls, movie theaters, or other buildings that have air conditioning. Stay in the shade rather than in the direct sun.

*Q:* When a cool environment is not possible, what else can be done?

*A:* Some simple things can help someone with MS to stay cool. Eat ice chips or drink cold beverages. A cold wet washcloth on the back of the neck helps cooling. Swim in cool water or wear a cooling vest. Two types of cooling vests are available. One has pockets in which you insert frozen gel packets, whereas the other contains coils that carry a coolant connected to a small refrigeration unit that actually extracts heat from the body. We at the University of Washington recently completed a research study showing that heat extraction definitely improves endurance and activities that require endurance in heat-sensitive MS patients.

*Q:* Why is low humidity important in maintaining core body temperature?

*A:* When core body temperature rises, the body normally turns on its own "air conditioning system," and air evaporates perspiration to produce a cooling effect. Lightweight clothing made of fabric that wicks perspiration away from the body aids in evaporation. More fluid intake is required in hot humid weather because the body is excreting more water through perspiration.

*Q:* How can you avoid overheating while exercising?

*A:* The key is to be able to exercise to maximum capacity yet produce a minimal increase in core body temperature. Exercise in a low humidity, cool environment so that the cooling mechanisms of the body can take effect, or use a heat extraction system. Follow the preceding suggestions for staying cool. Symptoms brought on by or exacerbated by heat associated with exercise will disappear when core body temperature returns to normal.

*Q:* What is the effect of temperature on emotional attitudes?

*A:* Impaired nerve conduction caused by elevated core body temperature can affect what are called "higher functions," such as memory, problem solving, and emotions, just as it can affect the function of arms or legs. Heat does not change the psychological makeup of a person with MS, but it can make the person depressed and angry about the effect the disease is having on life. A health care professional who is skilled in assessing and managing psychological problems, such as a psychologist, psychiatrist, or psychological social worker, can determine the cause of behavior changes and the best treatment possible.

*Q:* Is everyone with MS sensitive to heat?

*A:* Heat sensitivity is common but not universal in MS. An occasional person with MS may even have what is termed a "paradoxic reaction"— he or she may actually do worse with cold. Many people who do not have MS do not like the heat either, but MS heat sensitivity of the type we are describing is unique to people with MS. Just like people without MS, some people are hot most of the time and others are cold most of the time.

*Q:* What is the effect of cold on MS?

*A:* Certain symptoms of MS seem to be more pronounced in cold temperatures. Swimming in cold water may make muscle spasms worse. Cool weather seems to be less of a problem than hot weather because it is often easier to keep warm by layering clothing. Also, cool weather does not induce the "heat sensitivity" that is so typical of some people with MS. Cold feet can occur as a result of impaired circulation when a person does not have sufficient muscle tone in the legs to assist blood circulation. If this is a problem, wearing wool socks or a double layer of socks is a safe way to keep the feet warm.

# Multiple Sclerosis and Other Medical Conditions

*Q:* How does MS affect allergies?

*A:* Multiple sclerosis appears to be what we call an "autoimmune" disease (see pp. 5–6). The immune system is incredibly complex, and anything that affects it has theoretic implications for MS. Certainly allergies, other infections, and other autoimmune diseases should be kept in mind when the immune system is not functioning optimally.

*Q:* What is the connection between silicone breast implants and MS?

*A:* Ruptured silicone breast implants have been reported to cause symptoms that somewhat resemble MS. Silicone does not cause MS but may cause other symptoms. The mechanism of silicone disease is not understood.

*Q:* What is the relationship between MS and insulin-dependent diabetes?

*A:* Insulin-dependent diabetes and MS are totally separate conditions, although both are believed to be autoimmune disorders. Corticosteroids have been used extensively to treat MS. One of the side effects of corticosteroids is that they can actually produce a diabetic state that requires insulin therapy.

*Q:* What can be done to manage vagus nerve damage from MS that affects the heart?

*A:* Unlike skeletal muscle, which requires nerve signals from the brain and spinal cord to function, the heart has its own built-in regulation and pacemaker. Multiple sclerosis can affect parts of the brain and spinal cord that control organs such as the lungs and possibly the heart. The disease does not directly affect peripheral nerves, such as the vagus nerve. Rarely, MS might affect some of the nuclei in the brainstem that control and are related to function of the vagus nerve.

*Q:* Is there evidence that smoking has a specific detrimental effect on MS?

*A:* Smoking has very detrimental effects on health in general. There is no specific evidence that smoking is any worse for people with MS than it is for the general population. Smoking causes lung disease, which impairs breathing. This may be compounded by chest muscle weakness in MS. Cigarette smoke adversely affects blood vessels, which may contribute to impaired peripheral circulation, coronary artery disease, and stroke. In no way is smoking good for anyone, with or without MS.

*Q:* Should people with MS get a flu vaccine?

*A:* People with MS should get an influenza vaccine, especially if they have some involvement of chest muscles that would put them at risk for developing pneumonia. A number of years ago some people who received the flu vaccine developed an acute neurologic disease called Guillain-Barré syndrome. Investigation of that incident found a defective batch of the vaccine. Although some older books caution against it, we believe that there is no convincing current evidence that the vaccine exacerbates MS or causes other serious problems.

*Q:* Why does it take so long to get over the flu or a cold?

*A:* These illnesses often produce fever. When the core body temperature is increased, conduction in the demyelinated segments of the central nervous system is altered and conduction blocks that impair neurologic function can develop. When this occurs, the normal healthy status of the person is impaired. During that time there may be some loss of functional ability, which may take a while to regain. Some people with MS may also have weakened respiratory muscles, and protective mechanisms such as the cough reflex may be weakened. It should not take longer to recover from an infection just because you have MS. However, your body's ability to "bounce back" may be slower.

*Q:* Why does an exacerbation often follow a bout of flu?

*A:* Influenza is a viral infection. It stresses the body and calls on the immune system to rid the body of the virus. The additional demands on the body's immune system can predispose the person to a worsening of MS symptoms. A virus may also trigger an exacerbation through an immunoactivation mechanism. Additionally, fever is commonly associated with influenza. Nerve impulses across demyelinated segments of nerve in the central nervous system may become significantly impaired, causing symptoms that are not apparent at normal body temperature to appear.

*Q:* Does MS protect you from getting other diseases?

*A:* It would be nice to think that MS brought with it some immunity to other major illnesses, but that is not true. People with MS can get cancer, they can have heart attacks, and they can get acute illnesses such as the flu. Maintaining your general health and participating in programs that decrease your risk factors for those other health problems is just as important for people with MS as it is for others. Following a low-fat diet, giving up smoking, and exercising are some lifestyle modifications that markedly decrease the risk for heart disease and strokes. Be sure that you regularly have the recommended screening tests to detect other serious medical problems at an early stage.

*Q:* Have any studies been done on the relationship between MS and ADHD?

*A:* To our knowledge, there has not been any research directly linking attention deficit hyperactivity disorder (ADHD) to multiple sclerosis.

# Surgery and Its Effects on MS

*Q:* What advice do you have for people who need to have surgery and will be receiving anesthesia?

*A:* Surgery is a major stressor on the body, and it is speculated that this level of stress can result in an exacerbation in some MS patients. The stress may produce an immediate exacerbation or one that is somewhat delayed, or it may have no impact whatsoever. The evidence is not conclusive. If surgery is necessary, be sure that your general health is as good as it can be beforehand. It also is necessary to evaluate whether corticosteroid replacement may be required after prolonged use of this medication for treatment of MS. Having surgery places stress on the body, and healing power is enhanced with increased levels of self-produced corticosteroids. Long-term use of corticosteroids reduces the person's own ability to produce it, so that he or she may not be able to respond safely to the stress of surgery.

*Q:* Will immobilization of an extremity following surgery adversely affect MS?

*A:* Immobilization of a limb following a major surgical procedure such as a tendon repair may result in muscle atrophy and joint contracture. The ability to bounce back from a period of immobilization is diminished in someone with MS. Electrical stimulation of nerves and muscles during the period the limb is immobilized might be helpful, and special rehabilitative efforts should be implemented after surgery.

# WELLNESS MANAGEMENT

There is very little information available on the topics covered in this section for people with MS. In this section we answer questions that relate to empowering people with MS to take control of their lives and maintain wellness. People who take charge of their lives and take responsibility for their behavior do far better than those who assume a passive attitude. People with MS should make a determination that they care about their health and make it their highest priority.

Exercise is important to maintaining wellness. It is not only a scientifically valid means of increasing strength in people with weakness—even MS weakness—and a means of stretching tight muscles and preserving range of motion of contracted joints, but also it helps give you a sense of well-being. Conclusions from recent studies on exercise and MS have shown that exercises of various types—stretching/range of motion, resistive/strength building, and aerobic/cardiovascular—all have important roles in the management of MS.

At one time, when very little could be done for people with MS, dietary management was held in high esteem as a therapeutic intervention by some physicians and many patients. Scientific evidence has not supported the usefulness of any particular diet for MS. However, healthful eating is essential. People with MS are not immune to the number one killer in our country—cardiovascular disease. The American Heart Association suggests that not more than 25 percent to 30 percent of our diet should come from fat. Sound nutritional principles include eating more complex carbohydrates, fruits, vegetables, and whole grains. People who eat right feel better—and that's not just emotional, it's physical.

# Exercise

*Q:* Is there a particular type of exercise that is best for people with MS?

*A:* The type of exercise that is best for someone with MS depends on the severity and extent of the disease process, as well as on age and other health characteristics. For example, a young, newly diagnosed person who is otherwise healthy may have essentially no limitations on physical activity and would benefit from the same types of exercise, and to the same degree, as anyone without MS. In more severe cases, in which MS has progressed and weakness is a problem, research at the University of Washington has shown that resistive exercise can strengthen weak muscles to some degree, and that the increase in strength achieved can be sufficient to noticeably increase function. In patients with even more severe disease, the best type of exercises might be stretching, in which the joints are taken through full range and the muscles are stretched, to preserve full range of motion. Of course, concomitant diseases such as arthritis might produce other restrictions on physical activity.

*Q:* Is aerobic exercise beneficial to someone with MS?

*A:* Absolutely. Aerobic exercises are conditioning exercises for the cardiovascular system. A person with MS who has the physical capacity to participate in an aerobic exercise program will certainly benefit. If it is possible to keep the body cool during the exercise, it is likely that even more exercise will be possible and more benefit noted. Some people may be limited by fatigue. Aerobic exercise will not alter the course of MS, but it may improve general health.

*Q:* How much research has been done on exercise and MS?

*A:* The National Multiple Sclerosis Society has funded some studies on exercise and MS. We know that exercise in someone without MS builds strength. It also increases core body temperature, which may temporarily worsen some symptoms of MS in certain susceptible people. However, it appears to be helpful for many people with MS.

*Q:* Are weight-bearing exercises that do not raise core body temperature helpful?

*A:* Weight-bearing exercises have a positive effect on bone metabolism. Standing in parallel bars can decrease osteoporosis and improve heart, lung, and kidney function. It is also good psychologically to be able to stand up and face people at eye level. One disadvantage of exercising in water is that the buoyancy of the water does not provide the full benefit of weight bearing, although hydrotherapy can be excellent for maintaining joint range of motion.

*Q:* Can too much exercise bring on an exacerbation of MS?

*A:* No. Exercise does not appear to precipitate an exacerbation of MS, although exercise that raises core body temperature may temporarily worsen symptoms. This worsening of symptoms will resolve reasonably soon after the activity is stopped and body temperature returns to normal.

*Q:* Are there specific exercises that will strengthen leg muscles?

*A:* Exercise that involves lifting a weight or pushing against resistance can produce muscular fatigue. In fact, in healthy subjects the most effective way to strengthen a muscle is to exercise it to the point of fatigue. Ideally, a DeLorme progressive resistance exercise (PRE) is done by identifying the maximal weight a muscle can lift 10 times, and then lifting 50 percent (50 percent max) of that weight 10 times, 75 percent (75 percent max) of that weight 10 times, and the full weight 10 times; 30 repetitions (reps) in all. The so-called "Oxford" system may even be better for people with MS. In this regimen, the full weight is first done 10 times, then 75 percent max 10 times, then 50 percent max 10 times. Some recent research suggests that the full weight 10 times may, by itself, be quite effective. The problem in someone with MS is that another type of fatigue—central fatigue—can occur and may interfere with the strengthening "muscle fatigue." Also, the level of force that can be generated in weak muscles in people with MS is reduced, so exercise may not be efficient. It is not uncommon, for example, for someone with MS to be able to walk a short distance without difficulty. However, walking a long distance may result in foot drop. It is important for the person with MS to get an expert opinion as to whether exercise, the adjustment of medicine to reduce spasticity, or the use of ambulation aids and ankle-foot orthoses (braces) to substitute for muscles that fatigue easily is indicated.

*Q:* Can someone with MS go beyond physical limits daily or periodically without harm?

*A:* Many people with MS will have some physical limitations. Certain levels of activities will be comfortable, beyond which there will be a feeling of exhaustion. There is no harm at times in pushing those limits into the range of exhaustion, although persistent exhaustion and fatigue can be detrimental.

*Q:* What is the optimum exercise for people who are barely ambulatory?

*A:* The first recommendation is range of motion and stretching exercises. Moving the joints through their full range of motion only once a day may help prevent the development of contractures, which interfere with joint movement and impair the ability to perform activities of daily living. Any resistive exercise—that is, moving a limb against a resistance or weight—might also help. A physiatrist or physical therapist can determine the most appropriate exercises.

*Q:* How does someone with MS know when he or she has enough exercise?

*A:* Someone with MS needs enough exercise to maintain cardiovascular fitness and muscular strength, but not so much as to become exhausted. That particular point is very individualized. Working with a physiatrist, physical therapist, or exercise physiologist can help each individual determine an exercise level that is appropriate to his or her current level of ability.

*Q:* What kind of exercises are appropriate for someone with numbness and tingling?

*A:* Exercises are really not used for treatment of numbness and tingling that result from damage to myelin in the central nervous system. Numbness and tingling can also result from peripheral nerve compression or impaired blood circulation, and specific exercises might help to alleviate numbness and tingling from these causes.

*Q:* Can someone who uses a wheelchair participate in aerobic exercise?

*A:* Much will depend on why the person uses a wheelchair and how much muscle function remains. Upper body exercises can be done even when it is not possible to exercise the lower body, but they are less efficient in providing aerobic conditioning than are exercises for the large muscles of the lower limbs. There are videotapes and other exercise resources that demonstrate exercise programs for people with varying abilities (see Appendix A). Consultation with a physiatrist, physical therapist, or exercise physiologist can result in an individual program that will help increase cardiovascular fitness, even if a person is seriously disabled.

*Q:* Can strenuous exercise hurt someone with MS?

*A:* Strenuous exercise in someone with MS should not cause harm. The question to be asked is how long the degree of fatigue that results from the exercise lasts. If the fatigue from strenuous exercise continues into the next day, cutting back on the exercise would be appropriate. Otherwise, it is good to continue exercise at the maximum level possible. A good rule of thumb is that it should not take more than twice as long to recover from exercise as it took to become fatigued.

*Q:* Is it possible for someone with MS to cross the line of too much exercise?

*A:* Of course, excesses are always possible. Someone who has fairly advanced MS and who is very motivated may cross the line into an area in which they are losing more than they are gaining from exercise. For example, theoretically, lifting weights with muscles that cannot achieve the degree of tension within the muscle required to increase muscle strength and produce muscle fiber hypertrophy may simply cause fatigue without beneficial effects. Yet there is recent evidence that some improvement in strength and function may occur, even in these muscles. Exercise tolerance may change over the course of MS, and the individual should be monitored and the exercise program should be modified accordingly from time to time.

*Q:* Is it best to exercise every day on a certain schedule?

*A:* Consistent exercise is required to obtain beneficial effects. Ideally, aerobic exercises should be done for at least 20 minutes three times a week. The time of day that someone exercises should correspond to the time when he or she has the most energy. Normal body temperature tends to be lowest in the morning and gradually rises to a peak in the late afternoon. Exercising in the morning, when body temperature is lowest, helps to prevent heat-induced fatigue.

*Q:* Should someone who develops tingling or shaking in the legs continue to exercise?

*A:* Tingling that occurs only with exercise could be a sign of elevated core body temperature or another problem such as nerve compression or peripheral vascular disease. Evaluation by a health care professional can help to sort out the cause of new symptoms during exercise and let you know if you should modify the exercise.

*Q:* What should a person do if he cannot move his legs or arms?

*A:* Exercise is much more than just lifting weights. Exercise includes such things as passive exercises, in which a therapist or family member takes a joint through a full range of motion. This can be done even if a person has essentially no strength in that limb. Without normal movement, muscles and tendons can shorten, which causes contractures, and ligaments around joints can stiffen, which tightens joints. Contractures and frozen joints can result in serious skin breakdown. Therefore, some type of "exercise" is desirable for all people who have MS.

*Q:* Is an exercise tolerance test on a treadmill necessary before engaging in aerobic exercise?

*A:* The purpose of a treadmill test is to determine the optimal and safe level of exercise before engaging in a vigorous program. Some people who have not exercised as they have gotten older may experience ischemic changes—reduced ability to get blood into the heart muscle—with exercise. This is dangerous because it may cause a heart attack. The treadmill uses an electrocardiogram to monitor changes in the heart with progressive exercise. A treadmill test is a good idea for anyone over 40 years of age who has not been exercising and who plans to start an extremely vigorous exercise program, or for anyone with any indication of a heart problem.

*Q:* Can someone with MS improve strength through exercise?

*A:* In order to increase strength in a muscle, certain characteristics of contraction must occur within the muscle fibers. Ideally, for the most efficient increase in strength, contractions must approach two thirds of the maximal isometric tension within a muscle and must be sustained for a brief period of time. That is a pretty stiff order for someone who has MS. To whatever extent an exercise falls short of that level of intensity, the degree of muscle hypertrophy that results will be less marked. Some increase in strength will occur, but it will take longer to achieve. Demyelination interferes with messages from the brain to the muscles telling them to contract, so muscle exercises and muscle building will be suboptimal. However, that should not be used as an excuse to abandon exercise.

*Q:* What should a person do when muscles cramp during exercise?

*A:* Any exercise that makes symptoms worse or brings on other symptoms is probably inappropriate or is being done incorrectly. Gentle, slow stretching of a muscle before doing the exercise is usually helpful in preventing cramps. Once a cramp has occurred, steady stretching of the muscle may help relieve it.

*Q:* What is the relationship between exercise and blood pressure?

*A:* With exercise there is a short-term, transient increase in blood pressure. In the long run, a healthy person should have a sustained drop in blood pressure as a result of exercise. Weight loss, exercise, and

sodium restriction are the major nonpharmacologic strategies for dealing with high blood pressure. They apply just as much to people with
MS as to people without the disease.

*Q:*   Should a stiff joint be forced during exercise?

*A:*   A stiff joint may be caused by a contracture of the soft tissue surrounding the joint. Sudden forcing of the joint beyond its normal
range can cause damage to the soft tissue in the capsule around the
joint. A safer and more effective therapy is a *static stretch,* in which a low
force is applied to the joint for a period of approximately 5 to 20 minutes to gently force the joint beyond its contracted range. The application of deep heat to the structures to be stretched can also help to
achieve a better result.

# Swimming

*Q:* Is swimming good for people with MS?

*A:* Swimming and water aerobics are very popular in the MS community, probably because they allow a person who is weak or has some ataxia to use the buoyancy of water in order to perform activities they could not otherwise do. Swimming and water aerobics are also strength-building exercises for people with more advanced MS, because moving through water produces a mild resistance, and resistance helps increase strength. A person with ataxia may be able to do things in the water that are not otherwise possible, because the resistance of the water decreases the uncoordinated movements somewhat.

*Q:* Can swimming get your heart rate into the target range and assist with weight loss?

*A:* Certainly long-distance swimming can increase your heart rate to within target range. Swimming laps in an Olympic-sized pool or doing water aerobics that burn calories in excess of calories taken in food will assist with weight loss. However, it would take a great deal of swimming to make a significant difference in weight. Swimming does tones muscles, which contributes to the visual effect of a fit body.

*Q:* What is the appropriate temperature of the water in a pool for someone with MS?

*A:* Typically temperatures between 85° and 88° Fahrenheit appear to be beneficial for people with MS. Temperatures as high as 92° may feel good and are excellent for people with arthritis, but a temperature that high may increase fatigue and other symptoms of MS. Water temperature that is too low may precipitate muscle spasms and cramps.

# Diet

*Q:* Do nutritional needs differ among MS patients?

*A:* Different people have different dietary requirements. However, the basic vitamins and minerals required each day are the same for everyone within the same age groups. The number of calories needed varies from one individual to another and is unrelated to MS. Someone who has a small frame and a sedentary job needs fewer calories than someone who has a large frame and a large muscle mass and does heavy physical labor. There is no evidence that people with MS need specific dietary modifications, other than recognizing that a person with MS may be less active because of the disease and consequently requires a lower calorie intake.

*Q:* What type of diet is good for people with MS?

*A:* Many diets have been suggested for people with MS, but there is absolutely no scientific evidence that any diet modification alters the course of the disease. Good nutrition is an important aspect of keeping your body in the best possible condition, and the U.S. government food pyramid is an excellent guide for the daily intake of various nutrients.

*Q:* Can a low-fat diet help people with MS?

*A:* Low-fat diets have received a great deal of publicity in past years. We know much about the adverse effects of a high-fat diet on blood vessels and its role in heart attack, stroke, and certain types of cancer. A

# A Guide to Daily Food Choices

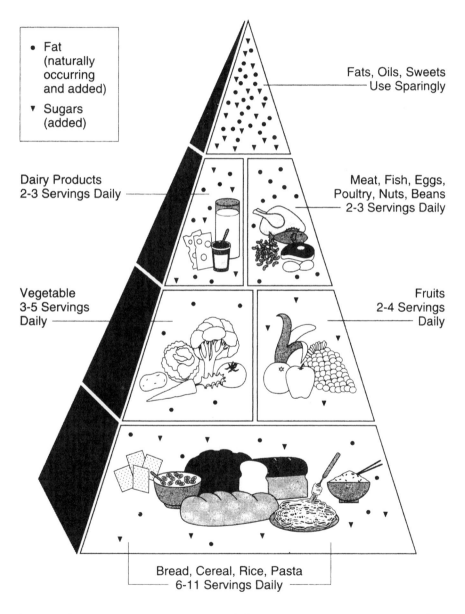

- Fat (naturally occurring and added)
- ▼ Sugars (added)

Fats, Oils, Sweets
Use Sparingly

Dairy Products
2-3 Servings Daily

Meat, Fish, Eggs, Poultry, Nuts, Beans
2-3 Servings Daily

Vegetable
3-5 Servings
Daily

Fruits
2-4 Servings
Daily

Bread, Cereal, Rice, Pasta
6-11 Servings Daily

*Source:* U.S. Department of Agriculture/U.S. Department of Health and Human Services

low-fat diet is not expected to alter the course of MS, but it is a health-ful diet that may prevent other serious illnesses.

*Q:*   Are there any controlled studies of diets in MS?

*A:*   It is difficult and expensive to study diets because it is hard for most people to rigidly adhere to a diet. There is much anecdotal information about people feeling better or noticing a change in symptoms with var-ious dietary modifications. However, there are no rigidly controlled, double-blind studies of diets for people with MS.

*Q:*   Can you recommend a diet that will give high energy and still help me to lose weight?

*A:*   Issues of weight loss are an ongoing problem, particularly for people who have a decreased ability to participate in activities that burn calories. Complex carbohydrates, which are found on the bottom level of the food pyramid, are used by athletes to sustain activity during marathon running and long-distance cycling. The portion sizes referred to on the food pyra-mid are quite small. For example, one half cup of most breakfast cereals constitutes a serving. A full and complete diet, but one that is low in fat—especially saturated fat—and calories is probably the best.

*Q:*   Can a diet take off inches as well as pounds?

*A:*   Generally speaking, exercise plus diet is more effective than diet alone for losing inches. A person who spends a lot of time sitting in a wheelchair or scooter often finds that the waistline increases in size. This may be due to weakness of trunk muscles and an increase in fat. Muscle weakness in MS can alter the type of exercise that you can do. The best approach would be to meet with a physiatrist, a physical ther-apist, or an exercise physiologist who can evaluate your strengths and weaknesses and design an individualized program that will maintain some level of exercise.

*Q:*   What is the best way to lose weight?

*A:*   Sustained weight loss is a long-term project. Crash diets may result in short-term weight loss, but dietary patterns do not change and weight is regained when the diet ends. Severe dietary restriction can result in poor nutrition and increased symptoms of weakness. Balancing food intake with calorie expenditure in a way that does not lead to feelings of deprivation is the only long-term solution to treating the overweight condition. A nutritionist can help plan a diet that includes your favorite foods, but is also low in calories and high in vitamins, minerals, and energy.

*Q:* Does it take longer for the body to digest red meat, and does eating red meat contribute to MS fatigue?

*A:* Whether to eat red meat is related more to its fat content than to the digestive issue. All of us find that we are a bit more fatigued after a heavy meal because our body's energy is being used to digest food. One way to overcome this problem is to eat lighter, smaller, and more frequent meals. Some people report that they do not feel well after eating red meat, but that is not specifically related to MS.

*Q:* Is there a connection between the ingestion of dairy products and the worsening of MS symptoms?

*A:* There is no evidence that dairy products have an adverse effect on MS. Many dairy products are high in fat, and fat is a health hazard. The use of nonfat milk and low-fat cheese is a good idea. In addition, some people lack the enzyme to digest lactose in milk products, but that problem is not related to MS. The symptoms of lactose intolerance are stomach cramps or diarrhea after eating milk products. Chewing lactase enzyme tablets before ingesting milk products reduces this problem.

*Q:* Have specific foods been implicated in worsening the symptoms of MS?

*A:* Surely someone has reported that foods ranging from potatoes to pork have worsened their symptoms! Although there are many anecdotal stories about the relationship between food and MS, there is absolutely no scientific evidence to support these connections.

*Q:* What is the effect of caffeine on MS?

*A:* Caffeine is a stimulant to the nervous system. Some people cannot start the morning without caffeine, and caffeinated drinks often get people through an afternoon slump period. Caffeine can be useful in helping to manage the symptoms of MS fatigue.

*Q:* Is sugar beneficial to someone with MS?

*A:* Fatigue that results from demyelination of nerves is probably not going to be helped by sugar. However, if a component of low blood sugar is contributing to fatigue, a candy bar may give you that extra push, although eating a piece of fruit is a much better choice.

*Q:* Why do steroids cause weight gain?

*A:* Two things may cause weight gain in a person who is taking steroids. Steroids affect the sodium and potassium balance in the body. Sodium is retained and keeps water with it, so some of the initial weight gain is due to fluid accumulation. This weight disappears rapidly when the drug is discontinued. On a long-term basis, steroids affect metabolism and may result in fat deposits in the trunk of the body.

*Q:* Can bananas help muscle cramps?

*A:* Muscle cramps in MS are unlikely to be caused by an imbalance of chemicals in the body. However, bananas and raisins are an excellent source of potassium and often are recommended for people who are taking diuretics that deplete the body of potassium, which may result in cramps.

*Q:* Do vitamins and other nutritional supplements improve the well-being of a person with MS?

*A:* There is no evidence that vitamin therapy alters the course of MS or improves well-being. However, we do know that malnutrition can have adverse effects on nerve and other tissues in the body. It is important for everyone to follow a healthful diet that is full of necessary and appropriate vitamins and minerals. Eating the recommended portions of foods on the U.S. government recommended food pyramid is an excellent way to ensure that nutritional requirements are met.

*Q:* What is the relationship between MS and vitamin B12?

*A:* Vitamin B12 is not deficient in people with MS. People who have an abnormality in gastric secretions such that they are not producing the intrinsic factor necessary for the body to absorb B12 have a disease called pernicious anemia. Pernicious anemia can cause neurologic symptoms that mimic MS and can be alleviated by vitamin B12 injections or the new sublingual vitamin B12 drops. However, MS is not benefited by vitamin B12 injections. Overuse of drugs that block the secretion of stomach acid can result in vitamin B12 deficiencies.

*Q:* How do herbal remedies help people with MS?

*A:* No known herb has been shown to alter the course of MS or to replace damaged myelin. However, a variety of herbal preparations have been suggested for managing MS symptoms. Some are a close analogue to pharmacologic agents and have similar side effects. The use of herbal medicine requires a knowledge of the herb's chemicals, its intended effects, its side effects, and its long-term effects. It often takes a lot of reading and talking to experts to get the necessary information about herbal remedies, with special attention paid to potential harmful effects or adverse reactions that may occur when they are taken with certain prescription medications.

*Q:* Is there any evidence that vitamin supplements affect MS?

*A:* With certain exceptions, vitamin supplements are not generally recommended for anyone who is following a well-balanced diet. Vitamins in pills may be metabolized differently than vitamins from natural food sources. The excessive intake of some vitamins, particularly the fat-soluble vitamins, can cause major problems because they are not excreted as readily through urine as are the water-soluble vitamins. Large doses of vitamin B6 may cause neurologic symptoms that can be confused with MS. A generic one-a-day multivitamin can provide insurance that all essential vitamins have been taken if your diet is not optimal. Additionally, you might want to consider a supplement of antioxidants—vitamins C, E, and beta carotene—but even their use is controversial.

*Q:* Have fish oils been shown to slow the progression of MS?

*A:* No. Fish oil is one of the many food substances that has been claimed to help MS in one way or another. Many people have testified that fish oil helps them, but no studies have demonstrated any real effect on MS.

*Q:* Should someone with MS take antioxidants?

*A:* Antioxidants may prevent the occurrence of certain forms of cancer. The best way to get adequate supplies of vitamins C and E and beta carotene is through food. There is less evidence that taking them as a dietary supplement is as effective, and there is some evidence that they may be harmful. There is no evidence of benefit in MS.

# EMOTIONAL HEALTH

The mind and body are integrally connected. Symptoms of MS can make dramatic changes in one's lifestyle. Coping with these stresses is a challenge for the person with MS and for family members. It often is hard to remember that you are still the person you were before you were diagnosed with MS. Certain personality characteristics help one cope with the disease. These characteristics include a desire to work at problems, resilience, and a belief in yourself. Developing effective ways to cope with stress is essential. Another important contribution to maintaining emotional health is to become a key player in your own health care by taking responsibility for your own life and your own body. Approaching the life changes that occur because of MS requires creativity. Creativity involves challenging assumptions, recognizing patterns, seeing things in new ways, making connections, taking risks, taking advantage of chance, and constructing networks.

# Stress

Q:  What is the effect of stress on the body?

A:  There have been many studies on the mind-body connection. Emotions and emotional health have an important effect on physical health. There is a close connection between the immune system and the neurochemicals that are produced in our bodies in response to stressful events. Ongoing stress places the body in a constant state of a "fight or flight" reaction that can have an adverse effect on the human body.

Q:  Should a person with MS avoid stress?

A:  Each person responds to stress differently, and different things are stressful for different people. Sometimes even things that are stressful at one time are not stressful at others. Although high levels of stress are not good for the human body, we cannot live in a totally stress-free environment. Researchers who isolated people and removed all stress from their lives found that without some stress people began to experience hallucinations and other signs of psychosis. The best strategy probably is to learn to effectively cope with stressors.

Q:  Is there a relationship between stress and MS?

A:  Certain responses to stress are not good for the human body whether you have MS or not. There are many reports and observations of stress increasing symptoms in people with MS. There may be no increase in symptoms during the time of stress, but an exacerbation may occur later, when the body's response has returned to a more normal level and the production of stress hormones has returned to normal. Several studies of people with MS have suggested that an increase in exacerbations may occur as a delayed response to stress. Although stress is assumed to cause a worsening of MS, during the Gulf War the level of exacerbations in Israelis under threat of bombardment from Iraq was actually decreased, again pointing to a likely "strengthening" factor of short-term stress. That being said, there is no acceptance by the MS community that chronic stress is good for people with MS—or anyone else for that matter.

*Q:* What are some constructive ways to manage stress?

*A:* The first thing is to recognize what things are stressful for you. Different things can be stressful to different people. It is most important to recognize how you respond to stress. Do you feel anger or sadness? Do your palms sweat and your heart beat fast? It is essential to know yourself and what works for you. Meditation works very well for some people, but for others sitting down to meditate increases their stress level. Exercise in the form of walking or working out works best for some people. Progressive relaxation exercises, guided imagery, or biofeedback can be used to learn how to relax during stressful situations. It is a good idea to sit down with a health care professional and talk about how you respond to stress, what kinds of things are important to you, and what activities you like to do. With this information a program of stress management can be developed that will help to manage stress appropriately.

*Q:* Does the diagnosis of MS cause mental stress?

*A:* For many people the diagnosis of MS itself can cause stress. Uncertainty during the diagnostic process is often stressful because there are unfamiliar tests that take a considerable amount of time. Many newly diagnosed people have never heard of MS and do not know what to expect. The diagnosis of MS may actually reduce stress because it explains the symptoms a person is experiencing.

# Coping

*Q:* What are the relationships between physical, emotional, and spiritual health?

*A:* Our bodies function as a unit; each part of the body affects the function of other parts. If we are under a great deal of stress and not coping very well, chemicals are produced in the body that cause sweaty palms, rapid heart beat, increased urine production, and diarrhea. When someone is managing a long-term illness such as MS, it is important to address all parts of their humanity, not just the physical symptoms.

*Q:* What can be expected of medical practitioners in helping someone cope with MS?

*A:* Many medical specialists have a role in helping to manage MS. A physician—often a neurologist or a physiatrist—diagnoses the disease and manages its exacerbations and progression. A physiatrist who is skilled in rehabilitation medicine can help maintain optimal function and activities of daily living. A primary health care provider will be concerned about your general health, not just MS. Psychologists help people work through coping issues. Social workers can counsel families. Multiple sclerosis and its effect on individuals and family members is complex. No one health care provider can be expected to meet all of your needs all the time.

*Q:* How can people with MS maintain a positive attitude when every exacerbation causes a more painful emotional crisis?

*A:* Maintaining a positive outlook on life is difficult when you have a disease that may exacerbate unpredictably and compromise your ability to maintain independence. One approach is to recognize the deficits but focus on the positive. Someone who is no longer able to run may give up by saying, "Now that I cannot run, I will not be able to maintain my physical fitness." Another approach is to say, "I cannot run anymore. How can I get around this? Can I walk? Can I do upper body exercises?"

*Q:* What role does a positive attitude play in someone with MS?

*A:* There is a close relationship between our physical well-being and our emotional well-being. Anything that maintains emotional well-being will have a positive effect on the body. Symptoms of MS will not be compounded if the body is in good physical condition. Keeping a positive attitude is one strategy for maintaining emotional health, but that must be balanced without denying what is really going on. It is important to use effective strategies for coping with symptoms of MS and not just saying, "I am going to think positively and everything will be fine." Having a support system or other people with whom you can talk about what is going on can go a long way toward cultivating a positive attitude.

*Q:* How can people with MS cope with the psychological stress that comes from others not understanding their plight?

*A:* One of the problems that occurs with MS is the "but you look so well" syndrome. Symptoms of MS often are invisible to other people. It is difficult to communicate the real effect that MS has on daily life. Someone cannot just look at you and see that you are fatigued or that you have pain. The National Multiple Sclerosis Society has an ongoing program of public awareness about MS. It is everyone's responsibility to help with that campaign. If each person with multiple sclerosis told five other people what it is really like to have MS, the awareness of MS and its effects would be markedly increased. Only when people begin to understand the diversity and mysteries of living with MS will they begin to respond appropriately to people with the disease.

# Mental Health

---

*Q:* What is the effect of depression on MS?

*A:* There are organic and nonorganic causes of depression. "Organic" depression is caused by MS-related changes to nerves in the brain, whereas "nonorganic" or "reactive" depression is caused by the reaction to having MS, but it is not caused by specific changes in the nerves. Depression and fatigue are sometimes difficult to separate. It is important for someone who has problems with depression to consult a health care professional who is familiar with these issues, especially as they relate to MS. It is important to determine how much of the depression is related to physical changes in the brain and how much is a response to stress. Understanding the cause of depression determines whether the depression is treated with antidepressants, with cognitive or behavioral strategies, or, typically, with a combination of both. We at the University of Washington and others are studying the effect of drugs on depression in MS.

*Q:* Does severe depression coincide with specific areas of MS demyelination?

*A:* It does appear that some of the depression and psychological problems that occur are related to organic changes in the brain. The National Multiple Sclerosis Society and other agencies are funding research related to these issues.

*Q:*  Is there any correlation between mood swings and MS?

*A:*  Mood swings are part of human nature. Some people with MS experience mood swings that are more pronounced than normal. Wide mood swings may be a result of demyelination in the brain or difficulty coping with MS. It is possible for people with MS to have concurrent illnesses such as bipolar disorder (manic-depressive illness). Anyone who experiences such mood swings should be evaluated by a psychologist or psychiatrist to determine whether the mood swings are a response to the losses and symptoms of MS or to organic causes.

*Q:*  What effect does MS have on personality and emotions?

*A:*  This is a complex question because demyelination in the brain can cause cognitive, personality, and emotional changes. A person's response to having the disease and his or her response to environmental, family, and job situations may also be factors. One of the major components in dealing with the psychological aspects of MS is the uncertainty of the future. Multiple sclerosis has the potential to be devastating, yet it has an unpredictable course. It can be very difficult to deal with this uncertainty. A counselor who is familiar with MS, its psychological component, and techniques for dealing with these problems can make a positive impact on the quality of life.

*Q:*  How important is a support group?

*A:*  Many years ago structured support groups were found helpful for people with MS. More recently, women who were terminally ill with breast cancer were assigned to usual care or to a support group. Those who were in the support group lived for years, whereas those who received standard care without group support died within a few months, as predicted. For some people, however, participating in a group is too stressful, and they should not be advised to do so.

*Q:*  Are the effects of support groups consistent?

*A:*  A lot depends on the structure of the group, the group leader, and the person with MS. Some people are not comfortable talking about any subject in front of a group. For others, a group that allows people to share their knowledge and help each other look at possible ways of coping with what is happening in their lives because of MS can be very helpful. It is not beneficial to sit around and complain about symptoms of multiple sclerosis and other people's response to the disease. A group needs a strong leader who can help people look at their coping strategies and develop problem-solving strategies for dealing with what happens in the group.

# DISEASE TREATMENTS

In the previous sections, we answered questions on symptoms and how they can be managed, as well as the management of health, or "wellness," in general. In this section, we answer questions on both conventional and less conventional therapies.

The decade of the 1990s has arguably seen the greatest advances in MS treatment come to market. There is great interest in the MS community about some of the new and encouraging medications that are now available. Three medications are now available for the purpose of altering the course of the disease: interferon beta-1b (Betaseron®), a medication given subcutaneously (injected under the skin) every other day; interferon beta-1a (Avonex®), which is given intramuscularly once a week; and glatiramer acetate (Copaxone®), which is given subcutaneously every day. All three are expensive, costing approximately $10,000 a year. However, scientific studies have shown beneficial effects of these medications in slowing the progression of the disease. Other medications are actively being studied along with new and innovative treatments such as bone marrow (stem cell) transplants. The future looks promising for the medical control of MS.

In the past, when no medication was available to alter the course of MS, many people sought treatment with alternative medicine techniques. Although we now have available proven medications, we believe that Western medicine should keep an open mind to some of these alternative techniques. They should be scientifically studied to ascertain that their use does not produce any harm and may indeed have some true benefit. For them to be deemed effective, they need to be shown to work; any improvement that occurs should be shown to be due to the treatment, rather than simply associated with a spontaneous remission or *placebo effect* (see p. 81).

# Drugs That Affect the
# Immune System

As of this writing, three drugs that have beneficial effects on the course of the disease are approved for use in patients, and other medications are in various stages of testing. Because of the rapid changes in this field, we provide more basic information on these agents rather than extended details concerning their clinical use. National Multiple Sclerosis Society recommendations are included in Appendix B.

*Q:* What is the length of time between the introduction of a new drug and its use in MS?

*A:* All new drugs must undergo *clinical trials.* Clinical trials are carefully conducted tests—usually performed in three phases of systematically increasing numbers of subjects—in which effectiveness and side effects are studied, with the placebo effect eliminated. These trials are difficult in MS for several reasons. First, the course of MS is extremely variable, and large numbers of people must be studied to determine whether improvement is brought on by the drug, by some other factor, or by chance. The second problem is the tremendous placebo effect in trials of medications for MS—someone may show improvement as a result of the sheer expectation of getting better. Third, bias may occur if the investigator knows that someone is receiving an experimental drug. The investigator may "see" improvement in the person that is really not there. Often the effects of drugs are small and difficult to measure. It takes approximately three years in a multicenter study before sufficient data are available to apply for approval from the U.S. Food and Drug Administration (FDA). The entire process to final approval may be lengthy, but can be speeded up if there is strong evidence that the drug helps and no other effective medications are available.

*Q:* What is being done to overcome the defects in myelin that occur in MS?

*A:* At present no drug is available that can compensate for the defects in myelin. However, there is exciting research in this field. Intravenous immunoglobulin (IVIg), which produces changes in myelin, is being studied as a way to improve conduction in demyelinated nerves. Digitalis, which works on the sodium and potassium pumps in nerve cells, may be helpful in improving conduction along demyelinated nerves. Other drugs such as 4-aminopyridine (4-AP) and related compounds prolong the action potential along the nerve and enhance conduction. Many agents that have the potential to improve nerve conduction in demyelinated nerves are now being studied worldwide. However, new evidence indicates that the nerve fiber itself—the axon—is also damaged in MS. Restoring myelin function alone would not be sufficient if the axon is damaged.

*Q:* Are the lesions in the central nervous system in MS as repairable as the nerve damage following a stroke?

*A:* Some of the recovery that occurs after a stroke is due to adjacent groups of neurons taking over the functions lost as a result of the stroke. A stroke is usually accompanied by swelling of the brain; when the swelling subsides, some or all function may be recovered. All of the recovery following a stroke is due to factors other than repair of damaged neurons. Multiple sclerosis does not generally involve such sudden damage to large areas of the brain or the resultant mass effect of swelling that is common in a stroke, so that type of recovery does not occur.

*Q:* If nerve cells are not repaired, why do remissions of MS symptoms occur?

*A:* An MS exacerbation may be caused by acute swelling of focal areas of the central nervous system. This can cause a conduction block in the nerves that originate or pass through the affected areas. Corticosteroids can decrease this *edema* and speed up a remission, stabilizing the blood-brain barrier to reduce an ongoing attack, but there is no actual repair of demyelinated nerve damage.

*Q:* Do methylprednisolone and prednisone help?

*A:* There is general agreement that these drugs should be used only for a short period during an acute exacerbation. Of the two drugs, intravenous (IV) methylprednisolone is safer and more effective.

*Q:* How effective is high-dose IV methylprednisolone in treating exacerbations of MS?

*A:* Methylprednisolone (Solu-Medrol®) is becoming the accepted treatment for severe exacerbations of MS. It is very important that the exacerbation be treated early. The drug is given intravenously in high doses (typically 1 gram per day) for three or more days and may be followed by a tapering dose of oral corticosteroids over two weeks. This protocol appears to be effective in reducing the severity and duration of an exacerbation. It does not affect the long-term course of MS and may not be appropriate for people with the more progressive form of MS.

*Q:* What happened to the use of ACTH for MS?

*A:* Adrenocorticotropic hormone (ACTH) stimulates the body's own endogenous steroids and is slightly effective in reducing the severity and duration of exacerbations, but it generally has been replaced by IV methylprednisolone. ACTH is not effective in altering the long-term course of MS. As time goes by, MS remissions tend to be less complete, resulting in transition to the secondary progressive phase and gradual worsening of residual neurologic deficits.

*Q:* Can the use of oral prednisone for another medical problem worsen MS symptoms?

*A:* The use of oral prednisone for any condition can cause serious side effects over time, such as alterations in metabolism, fluid retention, cataracts, and loss of bone mineral. The adverse effects of long-term steroid therapy must be balanced with its therapeutic effects. There is some evidence that the continuous use of oral prednisone in MS may actually increase the progression of disability.

*Q:* What are immunoglobulins, and how are they related to plasma-pheresis?

*A:* Immunoglobulins are antibodies that circulate in the blood. In some cases, they can be "toxic." Plasmapheresis is a technique that removes the toxic antibodies from the blood. It is being studied in MS.

*Q:* What cancer drugs are used to treat MS?

*A:* A number of chemotherapeutic agents that are used to treat cancer have also been tried in MS. The most commonly used agents are azathioprine (Imuran®), cyclophosphamide (Cytoxan®), and methotrexate. As a class, anticancer drugs appear to have a slight beneficial effect on MS, but unfortunately they depress the entire immune system, which then makes the person vulnerable to infections. These drugs also may have other undesirable side effects such as hair loss, heart toxicity, and stomach problems. Because they suppress the immune system, they may predispose a patient to urinary tract infection, which may in itself make the symptoms of MS worse. One primary new drug—mitoxantrone (Novantrone®)—appears to have more beneficial effect, but with less toxicity than some of the other drugs in this class. At the time of this writing, the drug is under review by the FDA. Newer treatments are aimed at modulating parts of the immune system without totally suppressing immunity. In some but not all people, they appear to slow the progressive form of MS.

*Q:* Are there any treatments for MS that are directed at the immune system?

*A:* Essentially all of the treatments that have been tried with MS are based on the knowledge that the immune system seems to be what destroys myelin. Interferons are part of the immune system, and drugs such as beta interferon have been used to modify the immune system.

*Q:* What is the drug 2CdA?

*A:* Cladribine® is the trade name of 2CdA (chlorodeoxyadenosine). It is an immune suppressor that is administered by an implanted catheter or by injection. A small initial study suggested that it slows progression in progressive MS, but clinical trials indicate that it is too toxic to be used. Many other drugs are currently being studied for MS.

*Q:* What has the study of oral myelin produced?

*A:* A multicenter clinical trial of Myloral®, an oral form of myelin, was started in 1994. The study was conducted at many sites in the United States and Canada, and neither the person with MS nor the researcher knew who was getting the placebo or who was receiving oral myelin. This is called a "double-blind" study and is part of a clinical trial. It turned out that oral myelin did not work in MS.

*Q:* Why does so much of what appears about MS treatment focus on beta interferon?

*A:* Two of the three FDA-approved medications are beta interferons: Betaseron®, and Avonex®. Interferons are part of the very complex immune system within the body. Beta interferon is an interferon (the "beta" form) that helps to modulate how the immune system responds. It reduces the frequency of exacerbations of MS and has been demonstrated to slow the progression of the disease as measured by MRI (magnetic resonance imaging). Multiple studies have demonstrated that the benefits of beta interferon—as well as the side effects of flulike symptoms—are related to the dose; the higher the dose, the greater the beneficial and adverse effects.

*Q:* Who should consider taking beta interferon?

*A:* Beta interferon is now approved by the FDA for people who have relapsing-remitting MS. However, a very large study in Europe has shown that interferon beta-1b (Betaseron® in the United States, Betaferon® in Europe) is also effective in secondary progressive MS. Currently there are clinical trials in the United States of the use of beta interferon-1b and beta interferon-1a in secondary progressive MS, and interferon soon may be approved by the FDA for this type of MS.

*Q:* Is there any evidence that beta interferons are beneficial for someone with progressive MS?

*A:* Beta interferon has not (yet) been approved by the FDA for use in either primary or secondary progressive MS, but a recent large European study has shown that Betaseron®/Betaferon® is effective in progressive MS. Your local chapter of the National Multiple Sclerosis Society can tell you where U.S. studies are being conducted (a summary of all existing clinical trials can be found at their Web site: www.nmss.org). Glatiramer acetate (Copaxone®) is also undergoing a clinical trial in primary progressive MS.

*Q:* What should I consider in deciding whether to use one of the currently available medications or others that may become available?

*A:* The National Multiple Sclerosis Society has recently published a recommendation (Appendix B) that patients should receive treatment with one of the "A, B, C" drugs (Avonex®, Betaseron®, Copaxone®) as soon as relapsing-remitting MS has been diagnosed. There now are many years of experience in the use of these drugs, along with many research studies. The data suggest that the most effective treatment— but also the one with the most side effects—is high-dose interferon beta. Interferon beta-1b is the highest dose interferon available in the United States at the time of this writing; a high-dose form of interferon beta-1a (Rebif®) is available in Canada and Europe.

*Q:* What are the side effects of Betaseron®?

*A:* Some people have a local reaction of redness and pain at the site of injection. Betaseron® makes some people feel tired and achy the day they take the injection. In most people the local tissue reactions and the flulike symptoms diminish over time. It is not uncommon for the white blood cell count to drop or for liver enzymes to rise slightly. Both of these abnormalities return to normal when the drug is stopped. We are learning new ways to prevent side effects and ways to help patients get past their early side effects.

*Q:* Will the cost of these drugs go down?

*A:* Interferons are produced by a very expensive technology using recombinant DNA. There is no reason to suspect that the cost will drop dramatically, although improvement in the manufacturing process and competition from other new drugs may result in some cost reductions. Neither is the cost of glatiramer acetate likely to drop much in the near future.

*Q:* What financial assistance is available for those who cannot afford these drugs?

*A:* Many people with MS have health insurance coverage that does not cover prescription drugs. Betaseron® has set up a foundation to provide the medication for people who cannot afford it. Biogen, the maker of Avonex®, and TevaMarion Partners, the maker of Copaxone®, also have financial assistance arrangements for drug coverage.

*Q:* How do the two beta interferons—Betaseron® and Avonex®—differ?

*A:* The two are very similar except for the dose, although there is a slight molecular difference, with Avonex® said to be somewhat more bioavailable per unit dose. Betaseron® (interferon beta-1b) is given at a level of 8,000,000 international units (IU) every other day. Avonex® (interferon beta-1a) is given at a level of 6,000,000 IU once a week. Recent research has shown that the effect of interferon beta on MS is dose-related; the higher the dose, the greater the benefit.

*Q:* Does beta interferon relieve the symptoms of MS?

*A:* Beta interferon does not have a direct effect on symptoms such as fatigue, muscle spasms, or the ability to carry out activities of daily living. By decreasing the number of exacerbations and stabilizing lesions in the central nervous system, beta interferon may prevent existing symptoms from becoming worse or new symptoms from appearing, but it will not reverse damage that is already present.

*Q:* What have we learned from those who have been taking Betaseron®?

*A:* Betaseron® was the first drug approved for MS in this country. It has been available since late 1993. Consequently, we have the most long-term data about it. A "phase IV" study has been collecting information from the thousands of people who are using Betaseron®. Experience has shown that people taking this drug still have exacerbations, but on average they have a reduction in the exacerbation rate and the exacerbations are less severe.

*Q:* How long will I need to take beta interferon or glatiramer acetate?

*A:* A reasonable analogy is that these drugs are to multiple sclerosis what insulin is to diabetes. As long as a person with diabetes takes insulin, the blood sugar remains under control. As long as a person with MS takes beta interferon, exacerbations should be expected to remain under control.

*Q:*   Can I stop taking beta interferon?

*A:*   We have experience with people who stopped taking Betaseron® and Avonex® because of inconvenience or side effects, or because it did not meet their expectations for decreasing exacerbations. The body does not become dependent on beta interferon, and no general adverse effects have been reported by those who have stopped taking the drug.

*Q:*   How does Copaxone® differ from the beta interferons?

*A:*   Copaxone® (glatiramer acetate, previously known as Cop-1) is not an interferon. It is a synthetic polypeptide that stimulates immune tolerance in the body. It looks like myelin (the "insulation" around nerve fibers) to the body's immune system and helps reduce the MS attack on the person's nerves. It is immunologically cross-reactive with myelin basic protein and may promote the development of antigen-specific suppressor T cells. It is a relatively simple molecule—four amino acids mimicking the antigenic portion of myelin. It is taken by subcutaneous injection every day and has been shown to be effective in MS. A major advantage is that this drug does not produce flulike symptoms. However, an occasional patient may have brief chest pain, which is worrisome but not dangerous.

*Q:*   Has there been any further research on the effects of gamma interferon?

*A:*   There are three types of interferon: alpha, beta, and gamma. Initially, gamma interferon looked the most promising, based on its use in patients with cancer. However, MS symptoms worsened in at least two clinical trials of gamma interferon. It is no longer being studied for MS. Interferon alpha is currently being studied and may be effective as a treatment for MS.

*Q:*   What does the future hold?

*A:*   One of the most intriguing new treatments is bone marrow (stem cell) transplantation. Because MS is an immune-mediated attack on the central nervous system, it would be logical to remove the existing "attack" mechanism. Bone marrow transplantation theoretically erases the body's faulty immune memory and replaces it with "cleansed" immune cells. This treatment is being actively studied at the University of Washington and, if effective, might stop the attacks of MS.

*Q:* What do you mean by a "placebo effect?"

*A:* A placebo is a "sugar pill"—an inert substance that the person taking it thinks is an active medication. The patient gets better because of the belief that it is of medicinal value. This can be a powerful effect and greatly complicates research on the effect of drugs for MS. Sometimes people receiving a placebo even report side effects identical to those of the active drug.

*Q:* How do over-the-counter antihistamines and other allergy medicines affect MS?

*A:* Antihistamines do not affect the underlying course of MS. They may, however, temporarily worsen symptoms of MS, including fatigue and bladder dysfunction.

# Alternative Therapies

---

*Q:* What do you mean by "alternative therapies?"

*A:* Any treatment that has not been proven to work in standard clinical trials may be called "alternative."

*Q:* Is there any indication that acupuncture is helpful for MS?

*A:* There is much about acupuncture that we do not understand clearly. It seems to be beneficial for some symptoms of MS, particularly pain. There is no strong evidence that it alters other symptoms such as bladder dysfunction.

*Q:* Is hypnosis ever used in the treatment of MS, particularly for anxiety attacks?

*A:* Many symptomatic benefits have been attributed to hypnosis, but it does not alter the course of the disease. A good operating principle is to look at the cost:benefit ratio. If it does not cost too much in terms of money, time, and energy to undergo hypnosis, it may be worth the investment to see if it helps relieve symptoms such as pain.

*Q:* What is known about shiatsu therapy and acupressure and their effect on fatigue in MS?

*A:* We do not understand the physiology of how techniques such as shiatsu and acupressure work. We *do* know that some people find them effective, particularly for treating specific symptoms such as muscle spasticity or pain. It is more difficult to treat a symptom such as fatigue with these strategies, although they often have a relaxing effect, which in itself may help lessen fatigue.

*Q:*   Can chiropractic therapy help symptoms of MS?

*A:*   Multiple sclerosis is a disease of the brain and spinal cord. From that perspective, chiropractic techniques have no place in treating the disease itself. However, chiropractic manipulations, physical therapy treatments, and other types of treatments directed at the musculoskeletal system may provide symptomatic relief of secondary symptoms of MS, such as contractures of limbs, muscle pain, and other musculoskeletal problems.

*Q:*   Can a chiropractor lessen strain on limbs that are affected by MS?

*A:*   The maintenance of health in a person with MS is a complex and interactive issue. People with MS can have the same variety of soft tissue problems as people without MS. People with MS may have decreased muscle strength, which makes them more prone to such problems as sprains, strains, and other types of soft tissue injuries. A variety of health care providers, including a medical doctor, doctor of osteopathy, or chiropractor, can lessen these problems. It is important to find a practitioner who is qualified and experienced in the specific problem and who understands MS.

*Q:*   Can massage therapy be helpful for a person with MS?

*A:*   Massage feels very good. Although it has no effect on the course of the disease, massage can help loosen tight tissues. It also increases blood flow to the tissues, and increased blood flow itself has healing qualities. Muscle tightness because of spasticity, inactivity, or other problems with MS can be helped by massage, and joint mobility can be improved.

*Q:*   Can massage therapy alleviate pain in MS?

*A:*   Massage is one of many therapies that work well for pain in some people but not others. The underlying cause of the pain is probably what predicts when massage will help. Massage has fewer side effects than drugs and certainly can be tried to alleviate pain.

*Q:* Do any studies with MS patients show an effect of visualization or autosuggestion on the immune system?

*A:* There have been many studies on the effect of cognitive therapies such as visualization and similar types of interventions on the immune system. Although we are not aware of any study in this area that has focused on MS, people with MS have been included in some of the studies. Those strategies do have a positive effect on the immune system and may be worth trying.

*Q:* What other effects do guided imagery and meditation have?

*A:* Guided imagery, meditation, and similar cognitive strategies are very beneficial. They help decrease the stress levels by altering how a person responds to stressors. These strategies are not for everyone. Some people do much better dealing with stress and improving well-being by running a marathon.

*Q:* Can biofeedback help a person with MS?

*A:* Biofeedback is most effective in teaching a person to reduce levels of muscle tension that are associated with certain types of pain, such as muscle tension headaches. Biofeedback also has been tried in MS with regard to managing spasticity or muscle tension. A number of studies looking at EMG biofeedback in people with MS have shown that it is less effective in managing spasticity than it is for pain related to muscle tension.

*Q:* What are the benefits of Tai Chi for someone with MS?

*A:* Tai Chi is a martial art that uses force in a therapeutic way. Martial arts will not prevent the progression of demyelination, but they have very beneficial effects on the body. Tai Chi focuses on the economic use of energy, strengthens cardiovascular capacity, improves digestion, balances energy and results in a dynamic feeling of health, and increases muscle tone, strength, and flexibility. It improves coordination, physical agility, and speed. Tai Chi helps to transcend internal or external obstacles, so it produces a feeling of focus in daily life, increased self-esteem, and self-discipline. Practitioners report harmony of mind and body, a positive attitude toward life and self, and a greater respect for self and others.

*Q:*  Are any studies of bee sting therapy for MS being done?

*A:*  Yes, and we should soon know if there is any scientific evidence of effectiveness. Bee stings have been suggested as a way to enhance the immune system in people with MS. Currently, there is no scientific proof that this is effective.

*Q:*  What is the benefit of hyperbaric oxygen (HBO) in MS?

*A:*  This is an interesting issue. A number of years ago an article in the *New England Journal of Medicine* suggested that hyperbaric oxygen was helpful in MS. Other centers tried to reproduce the effect and were unable to obtain benefit. For example, we did a study on HBO in which we measured such things as the ability of a person to walk in a straight line, the ability to walk quickly, and hand function, using a variety of measurements. We initially were very impressed with the benefits of HBO, but the problem was that people learned how to take the test— they simply got better at taking the evaluating test by retaking it! This makes MS research very difficult. The current medical opinion is that hyperbaric oxygen is not effective in MS and does not have a role in its treatment.

*Q:*  Are scientists studying treatment options such as evening primrose oil, flax seed oil, or Lorenzo's oil?

*A:*  Many, many treatments that are thought to be capable of altering the immune system have been suggested for MS. Not much research has been done on these substances as treatments for MS. Although some people have anecdotally reported improvement, it is not possible to sort out how much change in their MS was due to the placebo effect. Lorenzo's oil is aimed at a metabolic defect and is not appropriate for people with MS.

*Q:*  Would smoking marijuana on a daily basis help guard against the stress and pain related to MS?

*A:*  The active ingredient in marijuana has been shown to decrease the nausea associated with cancer chemotherapy. There also have been anecdotal reports of marijuana decreasing spasticity. However, small doses of marijuana impair the performance of simple motor tasks, reactions times, and short-term memory. Driving performance has been shown to be impaired for four to eight hours after marijuana use. Chronic use of marijuana has been implicated in decreased motivation, loss of effectiveness, impaired judgment, concentration, memory, and communication skills, as well as an inability to set goals and manage stress. The use of marijuana is illegal in many parts of the United States and may result in additional neurologic symptoms.

# Health Care Team

*Q:* When should a person consult a physical therapist?

*A:* Early in the course of MS, a physical therapist can help design an exercise program that is specific to an individual's needs. Even people with minimal disability can benefit from suggestions about physical activity. It is best not to wait until symptoms are severe before getting help. Reevaluation by a physical therapist is appropriate when there has been a change in functional ability and a new activity or exercise program may be indicated.

*Q:* Are there any specialized training or credentialing standards for physical therapists who treat people with MS?

*A:* Physical therapy schools are increasingly recognizing the important role that physical therapy has in the management of people with MS, and physical therapists are active participants in such organizations as the Consortium of Multiple Sclerosis Centers. There are increasing numbers of postgraduate and continuing education programs for therapists to learn about MS. However, there are no credentialing standards specific for MS.

*Q:* Does the National Multiple Sclerosis Society have guidelines for physical therapists who care for people with MS?

*A:* The NMSS does not have specific guidelines for physical therapists. However, the NMSS is very concerned about providing necessary information for people with MS. They have educational materials on exercise in MS that have been reviewed and approved by experts. However, caution is necessary in applying these materials because what is good for one person may be too much or too vigorous for another. Exercise must be individualized for each person.

*Q:*  Who should be included on a health care team for someone with MS?

*A:*  The person with MS is a critical part of the health care team and needs to be involved in planning management strategies. The signs and symptoms of MS dictate who else is needed on the team. Certainly someone who can take care of your general health is essential. This might be a primary care physician, an internist, or a nurse practitioner. A neurologist or MS specialist may be needed to manage the medical treatment and acute exacerbations of MS. A counselor, psychologist, or psychiatrist can help the person with MS and his or her family members to cope with depression or cognitive problems of MS. A physiatrist and physical therapist can address problems of physical function and activities of daily living. An occupational therapist, a vocational counselor, and a speech pathologist are also important members of the health care team. A urologist or nurse specialist can address bladder problems. A social worker can identify available resources to help the person with MS. Each health care team needs to be individualized and may draw on a wide variety of specialists.

*Q:*  How can people in rural areas contact specialists in MS?

*A:*  There are a number of MS centers in the country, and many are associated with schools of medicine that can provide consultation to physicians in rural areas. Your local chapter of the National Multiple Sclerosis Society can identify the nearest resources. Most large MS centers are members of the Consortium of MS Centers (CMSC).

*Q:*  How can someone with MS be certain of receiving quality health care?

*A:*  The person with MS is truly the expert in the effect that the disease is having on him or her and with respect to what things help and do not help. The National Multiple Sclerosis Society publishes newsletters and literature that bring people up to date about current treatments for the disease itself and its symptoms. The Internet has become a good source of information about MS. It is important that each individual with MS be informed about the disease and bring information as well as questions to health care professionals. The most important question to be answered is whether MS and its symptoms are being addressed adequately and comprehensively by the health care providers and the person with MS.

# SOCIAL ASPECTS

Multiple sclerosis does not occur in a vacuum. It occurs in the brain and spinal cord of people who have families, friends, and jobs. The way in which MS affects a person with the disease will have a major impact on his or her interaction with the people encountered in day-to-day activities. Multiple sclerosis is twice as common in women as in men, and it is most common in young women of childbearing age. The impact of MS on pregnancy and the effect of pregnancy on MS are ongoing topics of concern.

# Family Relationships

*Q:* What advice do you have for family members who are dealing with MS?

*A:* Multiple sclerosis is truly a disease that affects all members of a family. Just as MS differs from one person to another, families also differ. That makes it difficult to make hard and fast recommendations to families. Probably the most important thing is for family members to maintain open communication about the issues related to MS, to be able to talk about those issues, and to jointly solve problems related to those issues.

*Q:* How do you go about involving your loved ones in an active wellness program?

*A:* Wellness is not a solitary activity. It is one that involves the other people in the living environment. People who participate in developing a program are more likely to participate than they would be if they were just told what to do. To develop a wellness program, you probably need to work with a primary health care provider who can address all aspects of health promotion and disease prevention. Diet, exercise, and sleep are just as important as screening for major illness. Developing a wellness program requires that everyone in the family talk about his or her priorities and plans to manage such things as diet, exercise, sleep, and stress.

*Q:* Why do people withdraw from someone who has been diagnosed with MS?

*A:* The issue of people isolating themselves from someone with MS, or any chronic illness or disability, is a real problem that occurs too frequently. People often isolate themselves because they do not understand what is going on; they are frightened because they cannot stop the progression of the disease in someone they love. Illness in someone close often makes people feel vulnerable to illness themselves. The person with MS who needs to change his or her level of participation in recreational activities may find that friends withdraw because they want things to continue as they had been.

*Q:* What can you do with family and friends who isolate themselves from you when you get MS?

*A:* A lot of what a person with MS can do when feeling isolated depends on the relationship with the other person before diagnosis. Communication is an important part of dealing with that. If you have never been able to communicate well, it will be even more difficult to communicate now that MS is in the picture. Meet people person-to-person on an individual level to communicate about MS and how it is affecting you. Reassure them that nothing they did caused the disease. Help them look at how they can relate to you as a person, not as someone who is sick or disabled.

*Q:* What will help family members cope with changes in lifestyle after an exacerbation?

*A:* Communication is critical in helping family members cope with change caused by MS. It is important for the person with MS to talk about what is different in life, what he or she is no longer able to do, and to negotiate with other family members about how those things will get done. Looking at how you communicate and having some dialogue and sharing helps family members understand what is going on. Many of the symptoms of MS are invisible—referred to as "hidden disability"—and family members are dependent on the person with MS to tell them when a problem occurs. Sometimes taking the opportunity to talk with other people who have a family member with MS or with a counselor is helpful.

# Sexuality

*Q:* Can the disease process of MS itself cause a decrease in sex drive?

*A:* The sex drive is a complex phenomenon. It is a state of mind that can be affected by many things, including self-image and emotions. Physical changes caused by MS can also affect sex drive. Multiple sclerosis can affect the nerve pathways that are important for the physiologic responses associated with sexual activity. Damage to sensory pathways can decrease or make painful previously comfortable sensations associated with intercourse. Muscle spasms in the legs can create problems, especially for women. Drugs used to treat the symptoms of MS can blunt the sex drive. Damaged myelin cannot be replaced, but there are many things that can be done to work around specific problems. A counselor can help work through the emotional issues that may decrease sex drive.

*Q:* Is sexual dysfunction in MS ever psychological?

*A:* A major contributor to sexual performance is how people see themselves as men or women. Feelings of attractiveness can be altered because of physical disability caused by MS. Sometimes people think that they cannot be a good sexual partner because they have MS. The belief that you cannot have a good intimate relationship tends to become a "self-fulfilling prophecy."

*Q:*   What resources are available to deal with sexual problems?

*A:*   First and foremost is open communication. Talk to your partner about what is going on. Self-help books that cover all aspects of intimate relationships are available. Do not be afraid to seek professional help from your personal health care provider or from a marriage and family counselor.

# Pregnancy and Menopause

*Q:* How does childbearing affect MS?

*A:* We know that most women with MS do very well during pregnancy, but they may have an exacerbation of neurologic symptoms within 6 to 12 months following delivery. We have no way to predict who will have an exacerbation after delivery of a child, but we *do* know that pregnancy has no long-term effect on the progression of MS. Pregnant women should not take beta interferons because there is concern that they may possibly be associated with a higher incidence of abortion.

*Q:* What are the chances of passing on MS to my children?

*A:* Multiple sclerosis tends to occur a bit more frequently in families of people who have the disease than in the general population, but it is not a genetically inherited disease such as muscular dystrophy, in which the chance of passing the disease to children is statistically predictable. However, there is a genetic predisposition that makes it more likely that people whose close relatives have MS and who have other, as yet unknown, factors will develop MS.

*Q:* What advice do you have for a woman who is pregnant?

*A:* It is best to be prepared for the worst case scenario, and to have some support systems in place before your child's birth is certainly good insurance. If you do not need those support services, great! Planning ahead ensures that you will not be in a panic situation trying to find resources that you need in a crisis. The most important question for each woman with MS who is considering becoming pregnant is whether she is physically and emotionally able to care for the child. (For more information on this topic, interested readers may want to consult *Mother To Be: A Guide to Pregnancy and Birth for Women with Disabilities*, Second Edition, by Judith Rogers and Molleen Matsumura. New York: Demos, 2000.)

*Q:* What factors should I consider in deciding to have a child?

*A:* This is a complicated issue for everyone, with some added features if a parent has MS. The course that the MS is following needs to be added to the equation about having children. Raising children is a difficult emotional and physical task as well as a financial commitment. Physical care of a child can present challenges to a parent with a physical disability. Asking "what if . . ." questions and preparing for the worst can ease the role of parenthood. "What if one parent is no longer able to contribute to the work of the family?" "What if a parent is unable to maintain full-time employment?" "What if a parent becomes physically or cognitively disabled?" Knowing ahead of time your options for coping is good insurance that, like all insurance, you hope you never need to use. The good news is that we now have medicine available that controls the disease, and it is likely that new treatments will be even more effective.

*Q:* Can the hormonal changes that occur during menopause exacerbate MS?

*A:* We do not have any evidence that the normal hormonal changes that occur during menopause exacerbate MS. However, many of the symptoms of menopause are not unlike those of MS. Probably the best management of those symptoms is hormonal replacement with both estrogen (Premarin®) and progesterone (Provera®). Estrogen helps to manage those symptoms by replacing the estrogen that is no longer produced by the women's body, and the progesterone decreases the risk of developing uterine cancer that is associated with estrogen alone. Although there are no available data concerning whether postmenopausal women with MS should receive hormone replacements, the increased risk of osteoporosis associated with reduced mobility suggests that this question should be discussed with your physicians.

# FINANCIAL BURDEN

We have said in the preceding section on social aspects that MS does not occur in a vacuum. It exists in a person who has a family and friends. Typically, the affected person also has a job. The disease can affect employment and, consequently, income.

Not only may MS have a negative effect on income, but also the costs of care have skyrocketed with the advent of expensive new medications. This can result in an economic "double whammy" for the person with MS. At the present time, the A, B, C drugs cost approximately $10,000 per year. Although insurance covers the cost entirely in some cases, in most cases insurance covers medications with a co-payment, which could mean that you may have to pay as much as several hundred dollars per month for one of these medications. A person with MS who is on Medicare has an even greater problem, because at the present time Medicare does not cover the cost of medication, although there are pressures on the program to cover drugs. This may mean that the person with MS who must rely on Medicare may, in reality, not have access to drugs that reduce the progression of the disease. For them, such a medication might as well not exist. Because of costs of medications and care, as well as the negative impact on employment and the long duration of the disease, financial matters are of great consequence for people with MS. For a detailed discussion of these issues, see *Multiple Sclerosis: Your Legal Rights*, Second Edition, by Lanny and Sara Perkins (New York: Demos, 1999).

# Insurance

*Q:* What can we do to get Medicare to pay for drug therapies?

*A:* Medicare does not currently pay for most medications. Contact your congressional and senatorial representatives and let them know the importance of including benefits for the treatment of chronic diseases such as MS in any new plans that are proposed.

*Q:* How has managed care affected the care of MS?

*A:* The purpose of managed care is to control health care costs. Committing to pay $10,000 a year for a single drug is not something managed care companies desire to do. As a result, many managed care companies will allow the purchase of medication only for FDA-approved uses. Many medications are used for "off-label" indications. These are indications for which the medicine works (or appears to work) but which were not part of the testing process (see the NMSS's explanation of this in Appendix B). Cost-containment efforts by managed care companies may involve disapproval of medications for off-label use. An example would be approving Betaseron® for secondary progressive MS, even though it has demonstrated efficiency in a large European trial, because the FDA has not approved Betaseron® for this purpose.

*Q:*   Is there anything that can be done to get insurance companies to pay for more physical therapy?

*A:*   Most insurance companies are willing to reimburse for short-term therapy programs when they can see measurable improvement. In a progressive disease such as MS, "improvement" may actually be a retardation of progression and the prevention of future complications. Write to your employer, insurance company, and congressional representatives and senators and explain your needs in terms of health care coverage, and why it is important for those needs to be included in new benefit packages.

*Q:*   What kinds of programs are available to help with the cost of medications?

*A:*   Many insurance plans, Medicare among them, do not pay for most drugs taken at home. Even when a policy covers a percentage of drug costs, the remaining portion can be substantial. Some pharmaceutical companies have programs that help defray the cost of their products. Berlex, the maker of Betaseron®, has established the Betaseron Foundation to provide medicine for many people who could otherwise not afford it. Biogen, the manufacturer of Avonex®, and TevaMarion, the manufacturer of Copaxone®, have more recently established mechanisms to assist in payment for these medication for patients who do not have adequate insurance coverage. Contact the manufacturers for specific information. Check with your health care provider who prescribed the medication for more information.

*Q:*   Will any insurance companies take on a person with MS?

*A:*   The issue of insurance coverage for someone with MS is a recurrent concern. Many insurance companies exclude preexisting conditions when writing a new policy. Some states have already made it illegal to exclude preexisting conditions. Health care and life insurance policies are available for people with chronic diseases such as MS. These policies often cost more because the actuarial data show that people with a long-term illness use certain services more than people without a health problem do. It is important that everyone with MS evaluate his or her insurance coverage. For details, see Laura D. Cooper, *Insurance Protection Planning: A Guide for People with Chronic Illness or Disability* (New York: Demos, 2000).

# Appendix A
## Exercise Videos

**"Yes, You Can!"**

ORDER FROM:
The MS Awareness Foundation
www.msawareness.org
4400 W. Sample Road, Suite 136-211
Coconut Creek, Florida 33073-3450
888-336-MSAF

**Keep Fit While You Sleep** (1992)
*Suggested audience:* People who use wheelchairs
(Note: film contains product advertising)
VHS 1/2 inch

ORDER FROM:
Twin Peaks Press
P.O. Box 129
Vancouver, WA 98666
800-637-2256
$29.95 + $4.50 handling

**The MS Workout**
*Suggested audience:* People who are ambulatory without aids
VHS 1/2 inch

ORDER FROM:
National Multiple Sclerosis Society
New York City Chapter
30 West 26th Street
New York, NY 10010
212-463-7787
$15.00

**The Wheelchair Workout**
*Suggested audience:* People who use wheelchairs
VHS 1/2 inch

ORDER FROM:
National Multiple Sclerosis Society
New York City Chapter
30 West 26th Street
New York, NY 10010
212-463-7787
$15.00

**Armchair Fitness**
*Suggested audience:* Range from people who are ambulatory to those who use wheelchairs
VHS 1/2 inch; 60 minutes

ORDER FROM:
CC-M Productions
8510 Cedar Street
Silver Spring, MS 20910
800-453-6280
$39.95 + $2.50 handling

**Nancy's Special Workout**
*Suggested audience:* People with MS, polio, spina bifida, etc.
VHS 1/2 inch; 45 minutes

ORDER FROM:
Nancy's Special Workout
P.O. Box 2914
Southfield, MI 48037
313-682-5511
$39.95

**Theracise**
*Suggested audience:* People with upper extremity disability
VHS 1/2 inch; 30 minutes

ORDER FROM:
Thera Cise, Inc.
P.O. Box 9100, Unit 107
Newton Center, MA 02159
617-332-6160
$34.95 + $2.00 shipping and handling

# ⥲ Appendix B ⥲

## NMSS Guidelines on Treatment— "NMSS Makes Recommendations"

The management of multiple sclerosis (MS) has been substantially advanced by the availability of the disease-modifying agents beta interferons 1a and 1b, and glatiramer acetate. A number of positive outcomes have been demonstrated in people with relapsing-remitting disease: reduction in frequency and severity of relapses by all three agents, and the reduction of brain lesion development, as evidenced by magnetic resonance imaging (MRI), by the beta interferons. There is also early indication of slowed progression of disability. After several years of experience with the beta interferons, and more recently glatiramer acetate, it is the consensus of researchers and clinicians with expertise in MS that these agents reduce future disability and improve the quality of life for many individuals with MS. The evidence for benefit from these immunomodulators is quite clear in relapsing-remitting disease. In addition, preliminary data from European studies of beta interferon 1b support the use of that agent in secondary progressive disease. For those who are appropriate candidates for one of these drugs, treatment must be sustained for years. Cessation of treatment may result in the resumption of pre-treatment disease activity with serious long-term consequences.

Clinical trials are designed to evaluate the smallest number of people, over the shortest period of time, at the lowest cost. In order to accomplish this, inclusion criteria are necessarily narrow. These restricted parameters of clinical trials are not intended to regulate subsequent clinical use of an agent. However, lacking clear direction, criteria for inclusion in the clinical trial often direct clinical use, necessarily limiting patient access to the new agent. With demonstrated benefit to people with MS from continued use of Betaseron®, Avonex®, and Copaxone®, it is critical that these therapies be made available to appropriate candidates early in the disease process.

The medical advisory board of the National Multiple Sclerosis Society has adopted the following recommendations regarding use of the current MS disease-modifying agents—Betaseron® (beta interferon 1b), Avonex® (beta interferon 1a), or Copaxone® (glatiramer acetate).

- Initiation of therapy as soon as possible following a definite diagnosis of MS and determination of a relapsing course.
- Patients' access to medication should not be limited by the frequency of relapses, age, or level of disability.
- Treatment is not to be stopped during evaluation for continuing treatment.
- Therapy is to be continued indefinitely, unless there is clear lack of benefit, intolerable side effects, new data that reveals other reason for cessation, or better therapy is available.
- All three agents should be included in formularies and covered by third party payers so that physicians and patients may determine the most appropriate agent on an individual basis.
- Movement from one immunomodulating drug to another should be permitted.
- Most concurrent medical conditions do not contraindicate use of any of these therapies.

# ⪢ Appendix C ⪡
## Foreword

*Multiple Sclerosis: A Rehabilitative Approach*
Kraft, GH, Taylor RS (eds.). Physical Medicine and Rehabilitation
Clinics of North America. Philadelphia: WB Saunders Company. 9:3,
pp. xi–xii (August) 1998.
George H. Kraft, M.D., M.S., Consulting Editor

Rehabilitative management of multiple sclerosis (MS) starts with stabilization of the disease process as much as possible and follows with compensatory strategies individually designed to substitute for lost function. In addition, MS rehabilitation requires attention to the unique needs of MS patients such as fatigability, heat sensitivity, and possibility of exacerbations. Management of MS patients is a challenge; no other disease has such potential for producing a combination of weakness, spasticity, sensory deficit, ataxia, and cognitive impairment—all with a progressive and uncertain future course.

Effective management can be structured using the following principles:

1. *Stabilization of the disease.* Since the early part of this decade, medical treatments have become available which have been proven to favorably alter the disease course. The first agent approved, interferon beta 1b (Betaseron reduces the frequency and severity of exacerbations as well as the progression of the MRI lesion burden. A second interferon—interferon beta 1a (Avonex) soon followed and most recently glatiramer acetate (Copaxone) has come on the market. All of these agents are effective in suppressing disease progression. These agents have only been approved for exacerbating-remitting MS in mild to moderate MS, but in June 1988, at the European Neurology Society meeting in Nice, France, in a large multicountry European trial Betaferon (European marketed interferon beta 1b) was shown to be effective in slowing the progression of disability in more severe patients who had moved into the secondary-progressive stage.

2. *Management of exacerbations.* Even though on immune modulating therapies, patients may still get exacerbations. These should

be promptly treated within four days of onset and 1 gram of intravenous methylprednisolone given for 3 to 5 days, followed by a week and a half of oral prednisone.

3. *Management of spasticity.* Spasticity is extremely common in MS and the clinician should realize that it is not always detrimental to function. In most cases it is and excessive spasticity should be reduced. However, testing lower limb stretch reflexes and increasing spasmolytic agents to eliminate spasticity is not indicated. Rather, it is better to test for clonus and reduce it to two to three beats, rather than eliminating it entirely. Because MS changes over time, clonus needs to be checked at every physician's visit and spasmolytic agent modified to produce the desired outcome of no more or no less than a few beats of clonus. This level of spasticity appears to stabilize patients' lower limbs; patients who have taken too much spasmolytic medication complain of "spaghetti legs" syndrome. Baclofen (Lioresal), dantrolene sodium (Dantrium), and the newest agent, tizanidine (Zanaflex), are all effective, but have different side effects. Severe spasticity of the lower limbs can often be managed with an implantable baclofen pump.

4. *True weakness.* Typically, this is first and most severely encountered in the lower extremities and presents an ankle dorsiflexion weakness. Testing for ankle dorsiflexion strength is best done after spasticity is adequately managed, since spastic plantarflexion can produce a dynamic footdrop, which will improve when spasticity is controlled. Frequently, stretching of the heelcord is necessary if preceding periods of spasticity have produced plantarflexion contracture. Management of weakness can be done in one of two ways.

> A. Mild weakness can be treated with stretching of the heelcord and treating ankle dorsiflexion weakness with resistive exercises. We have recently studied this and found that a three-time per week standard progressive resistive (PRE) program can be effective at increasing strength and function in paretic MS muscles. Occasionally, an MS patient who has been sent for bracing of the ankle will be able to walk unbraced with man-

agement of spasticity, stretching of the heelcord, and strengthening of ankle dorsiflexion.

   B. Moderate weakness requires orthotic management. Because of the tendency for spasticity and clonus and the need to provide a medial-lateral stability with appropriate cosmesis, a plastic ankle-foot-orthosis (PAFO) is the orthosis of choice.

The appropriate use of a cane is also used in conjunction with the exercise and/or orthotic management program.

5. *Management of fatigue and severe weakness.* Fatigue can be a major problem in MS. Pharmacologic treatment includes amantadine (Symmetrel) and pemoline (Cylert). Many patients who can satisfactorily ambulate short distances with orthotic management will need a wheelchair for long-distance ambulation. An electric scooter is commonly used in the MS population, because of the frequent coexistence of weakness and ataxia. Manual wheelchairs can also enhance function for some patients. To improve general health, appropriately prescribed aerobic exercises have proven beneficial.

6. *Heat sensitivity.* One of the unique characteristics of MS is that many patients adversely respond to increased environmental or body temperatures. When a urinary tract infection occurs, for example, producing a fever, patients often have a marked increase in spasticity and weakness. In our research, we have demonstrated that heat extraction using commercially available heat exchange cooling systems improves patients' functional performance. In addition, high environmental temperatures need to be avoided.

7. *Bladder management.* Bladder problems are frequent and typically consist of spastic or mixed patterns. In-office, noninvasive ultrasound measurement of bladder residual can be helpful in confirming the diagnosis. Small doses of oxybutynin (Ditropan) can be empirically used to manage many of these patients, but in more complex or refractory patients, urodynamic studies can identify the specific treatments that need to be employed.

8. *Emotional and cognitive problems.* Depression appears to be a frequent occurrence in MS and recent studies suggest that antidepressants (e.g., Prozac or Zoloft) are a very practical way of addressing this problem. Much of the depression may have an organic basis. Multiple sclerosis, especially in advanced stages, can take a cognitive toll on MS patients. Memory may be impaired and substitution techniques such as memory books can be employed.

9. *Other problems.* Because of the variability and extent of MS lesions, patients may have other problems, some of which can be very difficult to treat. Ataxia and intention tremor can be especially difficult to manage; no pharmacologic or surgical technique has been proven to be effective in the long run. MS patients in more advanced stages of disease can be subject to skin breakdown and, because of the inherent spasticity of the disease, severe contractures. Often by this stage, the disease is compounded by severe cognitive impairment as well. Such patients represent a management challenge.

The encouraging aspects about treating MS in the late twentieth century is that disease stabilizing agents, although not complete effective, are at least now available. With their use, it is anticipated there will be slower disease progression and less likelihood of MS patients entering the more severe phase of the disease. Rehabilitative techniques will occupy an important place in the management of MS for some time to come.

# ⁂ Appendix D ⁂
## Additional Readings

*Note: Your local chapter of the National Multiple Sclerosis Society has a complete collection of booklets and articles about all aspects of MS research, treatment, and management. Call 1-800-FIGHT MS to be connected to the chapter nearest you. Chapter personnel are available to answer your questions and send you information on any MS-related topics that are of interest to you.*

Barret S, Jarvix WT (eds.). *The health robbers: A close look at quackery in America.* Buffalo: Prometheus Books, 1993.

Bondo BE. *Tax options and strategies: A state-by-state guide for persons with disabilities, senior citizens, and their families.* New York: Demos, 1995.

Burstein E. Legwork: *An inspiring journey through a chronic illness.* New York: Simon & Schuster, 1994.

Cassileth BR. *The alternative medicine handbook.* New York: WW Norton, 1998.

Cohen MD. *Dirty details: The days and nights of a well spouse.* Philadelphia: Temple University Press, 1996.

Cooke M, Putman E. *Ways you can help: Creative, practical suggestions for family and friends of patients and caregivers.* New York: Warner Books, 1996.

Cristall B. *Coping when a parent has multiple sclerosis.* New York: Rosen Publishing, 1992 (written for teens).

Enders A, Hall M. *Assistive technology sourcebook.* Washington, DC: Resna Press, 1990.

Garee B (ed.). *Parenting: Tips from parents (who happen to have a disability) on raising children.* Bloomington, IL: Accent Press, 1989.

Giffels JJ. *Clinical trials: What you should know before volunteering to be a research subject.* New York: Demos, 1996.

Halligan F. *The art of coping.* New York: Crossroad, 1995.

Halper J, Holland N (eds.). *Comprehensive nursing care in multiple sclerosis.* New York: Demos, 1996.

Hecker H. *Travel for the disabled: A handbook of travel resources and 500 worldwide access guide.* Vancouver, WA: Twin Peaks Press, 1995.

Holland N, Halper J (eds.). *Multiple sclerosis: A self-care guide to wellness.* Washington, DC: Paralyzed Veterans of America, 1998.

Holland N, Murray TJ, Reingold SC. *Multiple sclerosis: A guide for the newly diagnosed.* New York: Demos, 1996.

James JL. *One particular harbor: The outrageous true adventures of one woman with multiple sclerosis living in the Alaskan wilderness.* Chicago: Noble Press, 1993.

Kalb RC. *Multiple sclerosis: A guide for families.* New York: Demos, 1998.

Kalb RC. *Multiple sclerosis: The questions you have—the answers you need,* 2nd edition. New York: Demos Medical Publishing, 2000.

Koplowitz A, Celizic M. *The winning spirit: Lessons learned in last place.* New York: Doubleday, 1997.

Kraft GH, Taylor, RS (eds.). *Multiple sclerosis: A rehabilitative approach.* Physical Medicine and Rehabilitation Clinics of North America. Philadelphia: WB Saunders 9:3 (August) 1998

Lechtenberg R. *Multiple sclerosis fact book, 2nd edition.* Philadelphia: FA Davis, 1995.

LeMaistre J. *Beyond rage: Mastering unavoidable health changes.* Dillon, CO: Alpine Guild, 1994.

Lunt S. *A handbook for the disabled: Ideas and inventions for easier living.* New York: Charles Scribner's Sons, 1982.

Mackenzie L (ed.). *The complete directory for the disabled.* Lakeville, CT: Grey House, 1991.

Mairs N. *Waist-high in the world: A life among the nondisabled.* Beacon Press, 1998.

Perkins L, Perkins S. *Multiple sclerosis: Your legal rights, 2nd edition.* New York: Demos, 1999.

Peterman Schwarz S. *300 tips for making life with multiple sclerosis easier.* New York: Demos Medical Publishing, 1999.

Pitzele SK. *We are not alone: Learning to live with chronic illness.* New York: Workman, 1986.

Pitzele SK. *One more day: Daily medications for the chronically ill.* Minneapolis: Hazelden, 1988.

Rao S (ed.). *Neurobehavioral aspects of multiple sclerosis.* New York: Oxford University Press, 1990.

Register C. *Living with chronic illness: Days of patience and passion.* New York: Free Press, 1987.

Resources for Rehabilitation. *Meeting the needs of employees with disabilities.* Lexington, MA: Resources for Rehabilitation 1993a.

Resources for Rehabilitation. *Resources for people with disabilities and chronic conditions.* Lexington, MA: Resources for Rehabilitation, 1993b.

Resources for Rehabilitation. *A woman's guide to coping with disability.* Lexington, MA: Resources for Rehabilitation, 1994.

Resources for Rehabilitation. *Living with low vision: A resource guide for people with sight loss.* Lexington, MA: Resources for Rahabilitation, 1996.

Rogers J, Matsumura M. *Mother to be: A guide to pregnancy and birth for women with disabilities.* New York: Demos, 1990.

Rosner LJ, Ross S. *Multiple sclerosis: New hope and practical guidelines for people with MS and their families.* New York: Prentice-Hall, 1992.

Rumrill, PD Jr (ed.). *Employment issues and multiple sclerosis.* New York: Demos, 1996.

Russell LM, Grant AE, Joseph SM, Fee RW. *Planning for the future: Providing a meaningful life for a child with a disability after your death,* 2nd edition. Evanston, IL: American Publishing, 1993.

Schapiro RT. *Symptom management in multiple sclerosis,* 3rd edition. New York: Demos, 1998.

Shapiro JP. *No pity.* New York: Time Books, 1993.

Sherkin-Langer F. *When mommy is sick.* St. Louis: Fern Publications, 1995 (P.O. Box 16893, St. Louis, MO 63105; fax: 314-994-0052—recommended for children ages 2–8).

Sherman JR. The caregiver survival series—*Coping with caregiver worries, Preventing caregiver burnout, Creative caregiving, Positive caregiver attitudes, and The magic of humor in caregiving.* Golden Valley, MN: Pathways Books 800-958-3378; Internet: http://www.caregiver911.com

Shrout RN. *Resource directory for the disabled.* New York: Oxford, 1991.

Shuman R, Schwartz J. *Understanding multiple sclerosis.* Riverside, NJ: Macmillan, 1988.

Stone K. *Awakening to disability: Nothing about us without us.* Volcano, CA: Volcano Press, 1997 (P.O. Box 270, Volcano, CA 95689; 800-879-9636).

Strong M. *For the well spouse of the chronically ill,* 3rd edition. Mainstay, NY: Little, Brown, 1997.

Tyler VE. *The honest herbal,* 4th edition. New York: Haworth Press, 1998.

Webster B. *All of a piece: A life with multiple sclerosis.* Baltimore: Johns Hopkins, 1989.

Wells SM. *A delicate balance: Living successfully with chronic illness.* New York: Plenum Press, 1998.

Wolf J. *Mastering multiple sclerosis: A guide to management.* Rutland, VT: Academy Books, 1987.

Wolf J, Miles M, Pickett K. *Vignettes: Stories from lives with multiple sclerosis.* Rutland, VT: Academy Books, 1993.

Wolf J. *Fall down seven times, Get up eight.* Rutland, VT: Academy Books, 1991.

ight LM, Leahey M. *Families and chronic illness.* Philadelphia: Spring House, 1987.

Younger V, Sardegna J. *A guide to independence for the visually impaired and their families.* New York: Demos, 1994.

Zola IK. *Missing pieces: A chronicle of living with a disability.* Philadelphia: Temple University Press, 1982.

**National Multiple Sclerosis Society Publications (212-986-3240; 800-344-4867) Booklets**

*Living with MS*—Debra Frankel, M.S., O.T.R., with Hettie Jones
*What Everyone Should Know About Multiple Sclerosis*
*Things I Wish Someone Had Told Me: Practical Thoughts for People Newly Diagnosed with Multiple Sclerosis*—Suzanne Rogers
*Research Directions in Multiple Sclerosis*—Stephen C. Reingold, Ph.D.

*ADA and People with MS*—Laura Cooper, Esq., Nancy Law, L.S.W., with Jane Sarnoff

*Enhancing Productivity On Your Job: The Win-Win Approach*—Richard T. Roessler, Ph.D., and Phillip Rumrill, Ph.D.

*Managing MS Through Rehabilitation*—Lisa J. Bain and Randall T. Schapiro, M.D.

*Food for Thought: MS and Nutrition*—Jane Sarnoff, with Denise Rector, RD

*Multiple Sclerosis and Your Emotions*—Mary Eve Sanford, Ph.D., and Jack H. Petajan, M.D.

*Taming Stress in Multiple Sclerosis*—Frederick Foley, Ph.D., and Jane Sarnoff

*At Home with MS: Adapting Your Environment*—Jane E. Harmon, O.T.R.

*Solving Cognitive Problems*—Nicholas G. LaRocca, Ph.D., with Martha King

*Understanding Bladder Problems in MS*—Nancy J. Holland, Ed.D., and Michele G. Madonna, R.N., M.A.

*Understanding Bowel Problems in MS*—Nancy J. Holland, Ed.D., with Robin Frames

*Moving with Multiple Sclerosis*—Iris Kimberg, M.S., O.T.R., R.P.T.

PLAINTALK: A Booklet About MS for Families—Debra Frankel, M.S., O.T.R., and Sarah Minden, M.D.

*Someone You Know Has MS: A Book for Families*—Cyrisse Jaffee, Debra Frankel, Barbara LaRoche, and Patricia Dick

*At Our House*—a coloring book for children ages 3–5 (contains very basic facts as well as an afterword for parents on how to talk to young children about MS).

*When a Parent Has MS: A Teenager's Guide*—Pamela Cavallo, M.S.W., with Martha Jablow

*Taking Care: A Guide for Well Partners*—Nancy J. Holland, Ed.D., R.N., with Jane Sarnoff

*Choosing a Pharmacy Service*—Virginia Foster

*ar Thinking About Alternative Therapies*—Virginia Foster

*Controlling Spasticity*—Nancy Holland, RN, Ed.D., with Serena Stockwell

**Materials Available in Spanish:**

Hacia una Comprensión de los Problemas de la Vejiga en la Esclerosis Multiple
Lo qué Todo el Mundo Debe Saber sobre la Esclerosis Multiple
Qué es la Esclerosis Multiple?
Qué le Interesa Conocer sobre la Esclerosis Multiple?
Sobre la Conservación de Energia
Sobre la Fatiga
Sobre las Problemas Sexuales que no Mencionan los Medicos
Sobre el Diagnástico: Atando Los Cabos de una Larga Historia

**Other MS Society Publications:**

*The History of Multiple Sclerosis* (reprint)—Loren Rolak, M.D.
*Facts and Issues* (reprints of articles that originally appeared in the National MS Society magazine, *Inside MS*, covering such topics as diagnosis, disclosure, pregnancy, pain, fatigue, energy management, gait problems, sexuality, depression, hiring home help, computer adaptations, genes and MS susceptibility, complementary therapies, etc.)
*Inside MS*—a 32-page magazine for people living with MS published three times yearly
*Inside MS Bulletin*—an 8-page newsletter for donors and friends (published three times a year)
*Knowledge is Power*—a series of articles for individuals newly diagnosed with MS
*Living Well with MS*—a series of workbooks written for, and by, people who have been living with MS for some time.

**Monograph Series (1995)**
*Families Affected by Multiple Sclerosis: Disease Impacts and Coping Strategies*—Rosalind C. Kalb, Ph.D.
*Long-Term Care and Multiple Sclerosis*—Debra Frankel, M.S., O.T.R.
*Employment and Multiple Sclerosis*—Nicholas G. LaRocca, Ph.D.
*Economic Costs of Multiple Sclerosis: How Much and Who Pays*—Carol Harvey, Ph.D.

*Utilization and Perceptions of Healthcare Services by People with MS*—Leon Sternfeld, M.D., Ph.D., M.P.H.

**Canadian Multiple Sclerosis Society Publication (416-922-6065)**
*Coping with Fatigue in MS Takes Understanding and Planning*—Alexander Burnfield, M.B., M.R.C. Psych.

**Eastern Paralyzed Veterans Association Publications (800-444-0120)**
*Understanding the Americans with Disabilities Act* (English and Spanish)
*The ADA: Resource Information Guide* (bibliography of books and video-tapes)
*Air Carrier Access* (defines the Air Carrier Access Act and gives information about air travel for wheelchair users)
*Accessible Building Design* (a description of the essential components of an accessible building, including dimensions)
*Planning for Access: A Guide for Planning and Modifying Your Home*
*Programs of EPVA* (a summary of fifteen programs designed to improve the lives of spinal cord injured veterans and people with disabilities)

**General Publications**
*Access to Travel*—A quarterly magazine published by the Society for the Advancement of Travel for the Handicapped—SATH—a nonprofit organization that works to create a barrier-free environment throughout the travel and tourism industry (347 Fifth Avenue, Suite 610, New York, NY 10016; 212-447-7284)
*An Approach to Barrier Free Design*—A magazine available from A Positive Approach, Inc., a nonprofit organization that services individuals with disabilities (P.O. Box 910, Millville, NJ 08322; 609-451-4777)
*Handicapped Americans Reports*—a biweekly newsletter that reports disability-related events and issues, published by Capital Publications, Inc. (1300 N. 17th Street, Arlington, VA 22209; 703-528-1100)
*Mainstream*—A monthly magazine available from Exploding Myths, Inc. (2973 Beech Street, San Diego, CA 92101; 619-234-3138)
*New Mobility*—A monthly magazine available from Miramar Communications (23815 Stuart Ranch Road, P.O. Box 8987, Malibu, CA 90265; 800-543-4116)

*A Positive Approach*—A magazine available from A Positive Approach, Inc., a nonprofit organization that services individuals with disabilities (P.O. Box 910, Millville, NJ 08322; 609-451-4777)

*Take Care*—A quarterly newsletter for caregivers published by the National Family Caregivers Association (9621 East Bexhill Drive, Kensington, MD 20895; 301-942-6430)

*The Very Special Traveler*—A bimonthly newsletter for people with disabilities who travel, published by Beverly Nelson (The Very Special Traveler, P.O. Box 756, New Windsor, MD 21776-9016; 410-635-2881)

*We Magazine*—subscription magazine published six times a year (800-WEMAG26; website: www.wemagazine.com).

*"We're Accessible": News for Disabled Travelers*—A newsletter from British Colombia for world travelers with disabilities (Lynne Atkinson, 32-1675 Cypress St., Vancouver, B.C. V6J 3L4; 604-731-2197)

# ⥈ Index ⥈